Fearlessly Fit

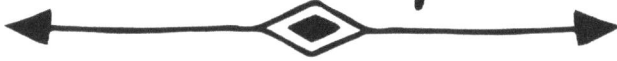

A 6-Week Fitness, Food & Faith Bible Study

Alisa Hope Wagner

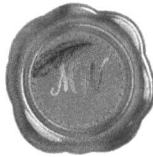

Marked Writers Publishing

Fearlessly Fit

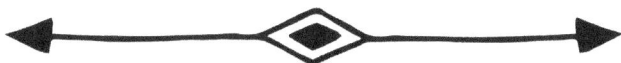

Alisa Hope Wagner

Fearlessly Fit
A 6-Week Fitness, Food & Faith Bible Study
Copyright @ 2015 by Alisa Hope Wagner.
All rights reserved.
Marked Writers Publishing
www.alisahopewagner.com

Cover design by Alisa Hope Wagner
Author Photo by Lori Stead of www.wetsilver.com

ISBN-13: 978-0692538975 (Alisa Hope Wagner)
ISBN-10: 0692538976
BISAC: Health/Fitness/Spiritual Growth

Endorsements

"Paying attention to the connection between the mind, body, and spirit is critical in social work. Alisa Wagner has written a comprehensive resource built on evidenced-based information that helps the reader understand the importance of food and fitness from a Christian perspective. I highly recommend adding this book to your personal library and to use as a recommended resource to clients."

- Cynthia Faulkner, Ph.D., LCSW-S, ACSW is a professor of Social Work at Morehead State University Morehead, Kentucky.

"Alisa Wagner's passion for ultimate health, both physical and spiritual, is evident in the pages of her latest book, *Fearlessly Fit*. Each chapter vividly intertwines the aspects of nutrition, exercise and scripture in a manner that encourages and motivates the reader towards positive change. Alisa is gifted with the ability to "spur" others on, making the reader feel as if she is right there with us on the path to attaining our goals by overcoming common barriers."

- Leann Minners, RD/LD (Registered Dietitian/ Licensed Dietitian).

"As a psychotherapist, I work with people who are struggling to find balance, peace and well being in their lives. As a team, we create a treatment plan to overcome obstacles and make changes that lead towards a happier and more fulfilled self. I truly believe that Alisa Hope Wagner's book can be an integral component of the treatment plan for many of my clients. The book is easy to read, full of important information, written in an encouraging voice and a must read for anyone struggling with food and/or inactivity."

- Christina Ketchum is a psychotherapist and Executive Director of Life Branch, Inc.

"In reading Alisa Hope Wagner's book, I was struck by the ease with which she conveyed the connection of health and well-being with profound spiritual truths. The WISDOM within speaks as God's Handbook to wellness. As a nurse, I feel she very accurately spoke of the complexities of treating the WHOLE person: body, mind, and soul... while connecting very personally with the reader to allow those truths to permeate the core. This book appeals to anyone in any phase of their health/fitness journey... and we ALL have one."

- Robin L. McNaueal is a registered nurse with over 18 years experience working with adult and pediatric patient populations in acute care settings.

"God has a plan for each and every one of us, and He has given us a tool to achieve it. *Fearlessly Fit* is an awesome tool to help its readers to start and keep living a healthy lifestyle. No crazy fads. The basic nutritional information, realistic workouts, and God's words give Alisa's book its title. Use this book to change your life."

- Faith Wilde has been certified for personal training through NCSF. She has been a personal trainer for 12 years, donating her talents to various ministries during her training career. "I love to teach woman that they can already lift heavy; they just need to learn how to do it."

Dedication

God—my Creator, Savior and Counselor

Daniel—my high school sweetheart and soul mate

Isaac—my first-born son

Levi—my brown-eyed boy

Karis Ruth—my cherished girl

Christina—my twin

I want to offer my sincerest gratitude to my family and friends who took the time to read my initial draft and offer me their valuable feedback. I'm blessed by the sacrifice of time and energy you made for this book, and I'm grateful for your encouragement and counsel. I pray that your work on behalf of this book will reap a harvest of eternal blessings. Thank you to Daniel Wagner, Patti Coughlin, Cynthia Faulkner, Christina Ketchum, Leann Minners and Robin McNaueal. I am honored by your words.

Also, I would like to give my earnest appreciation to the readers of this book. Many times God brings us to a point of transition in our lives, and there is always a struggle to grow and stretch with the changes that He has ordained for us. This struggle doesn't mean we are failing; rather, it shows that we are making the effort to transform into a better version of ourselves. I pray that this book empowers the readers on their quest to transform and improve their health. I know the journey will be difficult, and we may fall now and again, but to fall a hundred times is better to have never started.

Further, I would like to thank *International Sports Sciences Association* (ISSA) for their amazing health and fitness programs. The Specialist in Fitness Nutrition Course and the Certified Fitness Trainer Courses have helped guide my journey to a healthier lifestyle. The insights provided by a great team of researchers and writers have proven valuable to writing this book.

Last, I am honored to have competed and placed in the *Texas Shredder Classic 2015 and 2016.* This is a family-centered, drugfree body-building competition that is founded on the saving grace of Christ. I am grateful for a competitive platform that is rich in integrity, commitment and hard work.

Forward

I see it every day. As an Emergency Medicine Physician on the frontlines of American healthcare, I'm exposed to diseases that prematurely end the lives of their victims. Many of these diseases are preventable if we just took action in the things we easily overlook. One of these is food. I believe that food addiction is as dangerous as drug and alcohol addiction. The effects of poor choices in food intake can be just as devastating as any other addiction. Diabetes, high blood pressure, high cholesterol, cardiovascular disease, strokes and cancer can all be rooted in unhealthy eating habits and lack of exercise. People ravished with these diseases become dependent on medication and often times live a much less fulfilling life due to their poor health.

Hosea 4.6 reads, "*My people are destroyed from lack of knowledge*" (NIV). Fitness and nutrition have a language and vocabulary all their own. Alisa Hope Wagner shines a light on areas of health that give the readers knowledge, encouragement and motivation based on Biblical principles. As with many other aspects of life, the spiritual component of health is just as important as the air we breathe and the food we eat. Alisa's breakthrough health book, *Fearlessly Fit*, will give readers the keys to living an unlimited life, allowing them to achieve their God-given potential. I encourage everyone to read this book and to apply its principles, so they may embrace the abundant life that God has for them.

- Daniel J. Wagner, M.D. is a board certified Emergency Medicine Physician who has been practicing medicine since 2002. He is co-owner of TLC Complete Care, providing world-class healthcare to South Texas.

Introduction
A Supernatural Battle

"Be alert and of sober mind. Your enemy the devil prowls around like a roaring lion looking for someone to devour" (1 Peter 5.8 NIV).

There is a spiritual battle raging against the health of the American people. Never before in our history has there been so many choices of unhealthy foods and sedentary activities. The enemy is aggressively trying to steal years from us and destroy our quality of life. Satan hates us with a supernatural revulsion that we can't even fathom. And he will do anything to knock us off God's greater plan for our lives. He wants us tormented by our weight and health, so he can stand over our shame and point his nasty finger at our face and mock the creation that reflects the image of God.

"So God created mankind in his own image, in the image of God he created them; male and female he created them" (Genesis 1.27 NIV).

The enemy's sole desire is to make us forfeit our full purpose and to distract us from God's Kingdom Movements. He knows that we have been **fearlessly made,** so he will use whatever means possible to force us to walk in a lesser vision than the one God has planned for us, and unhealthy food choices and lack of fitness are turning out to be great tools for the enemy. He's laughing as we fill our bellies with nutritionally bankrupt foods and sedating our body with motionless activities because the enemy knows eventually those seemingly insignificant choices will land us straight onto a hospital bed.

Chronic diseases due to lifestyle choices—relating to our food consumption and activity level—are on the rise, costing Americans money, quality of life, their God-given destiny and valuable years on earth. Obesity-related illnesses include heart disease, stroke, type 2 diabetes and certain types of cancer. These chronic diseases are some of the leading causes of preventable death. According to the Centers for Disease Control and Prevention in 2025:

Two out of five adults are defined as obese, and six out of ten adults have a chronic disease.

Seven of the ten leading causes of death are due to chronic disease.

More than three out of four adults don't get the recommended amount of exercise, and fewer than one in ten eat the recommended amount of fruits and vegetables.

Eighty-four percent of all health care costs go to help people suffering from chronic disease.

Many factors contributing to chronic diseases are **preventable**. Because of the rise of sedentary activities and the production of high caloric, low nutritional foods, America's weight is ballooning every year. Gaining knowledge and implementing simple lifestyle changes will **revolutionize** our health, preventing a poor quality of life that relies heavily on medical intervention. **Awareness to this epidemic is the first key to fighting it**. Once we realize the magnitude of what's happening to us, we can arm ourselves with the knowledge we need to overcome and triumph.

"I praise you because I am fearfully and wonderfully made; your works are wonderful, I know that full well" (Psalm 139.14 NIV).

Although these statistics show a very dangerous trend in America, we should take heart. We can be *fearlessly fit* because we have been *fearfully made*.

And there is good news. There is One who has overcome all of Satan's wryly schemes—Jesus.

"I have told you these things, so that in me you may have peace. In this world you will have trouble. But take heart. I have overcome the world" (John 16.33 NIV).

Jesus said that we would have troubles in this life, and He knew that our current generation would be facing the *Great Battle of the Bulge*. God has not given up on us, and He understands that with a few key changes in our lifestyle, we can break the stronghold of weight that's holding us back.

*"Therefore, since we are surrounded by so great a cloud of witnesses, let us also **lay aside every weight**, and sin which clings so closely, and let us run with endurance the race that is set before us" (Hebrews 12.1 ESV).*

God wants us to feel good about ourselves, so we can accomplish the great things that He had planned for us. He knows that it's difficult to stay focused on the things above when we're not even comfortable in our own skin. God will give us the strength to claim not just a healthy lifestyle, but a FEARLESS lifestyle.

God designed our body: they are resilient, strong and easily transformed. Let's give Him our willingness to start experiencing our fitness, food and faith victory today. We can be fearlessly fit, knowing that if God is with us, we have nothing to fear.

"What, then, shall we say in response to these things? If God is for us, who can be against us?" (Romans 8.31 NIV).

As we continue on the health experience, we will need to download a calorie counter app. This app will help alleviate the guesswork of calorie counting and will speed up the process.

Chapter 1

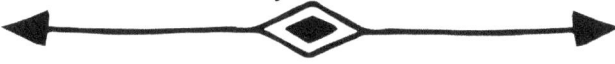

"Do you not know that you are God's temple and that God's Spirit dwells in you? If anyone destroys God's temple, God will destroy him. For God's temple is holy, and you are that temple" (1 Corinthians 3.16-17 ESV).

Fitness
Three Body Types

God's Children were created equal, but we weren't created the same. Although the current pop media would like to give us their cookie-cutter version of the perfect body, our culture's idealized physique is not possible for most people; in fact, this version of a "perfect" body is an image of unhealthiness for many individuals. God has created each of us uniquely and beautifully, and nothing He creates is by mistake. Once we embrace our own body, we will see it as the masterpiece that it is and treat it with respect.

"For we are God's masterpiece. He has created us anew in Christ Jesus, so we can do the good things he planned for us long ago" (Ephesians 2.10 NLT).

The first thing we need to do is stop comparing ourselves to others. This is the surest way to steal our peace and contentment with the body God has given us. We only have our body for a short period of time on this earth, so we NEED to embrace it and take care of it as good stewards of the Lord. Our body is aging every day, so we might as well enjoy each season of life that we are blessed to experience.

*"Each one should test their own actions. Then they can take pride in themselves alone, **without comparing themselves to someone else**" (Galatians 6.4 NIV).*

From a distance anyone can look perfect, but the truth is that each one of us has things we like and dislike about our body, and we must take the good with the bad. After we come to terms with our personal body issues, we will realize that our flaws are not such a big deal. In light of God's goodness and love, all of our body image strongholds will pale in comparison.

There are three main body types found in the human race. Although, many of us will be a mix of two of them, we will favor one body type the most. Once we know our personal body type, we can gain more tangible health and fitness goals and expectations.

Ectomorphs –These people have a thin build with long and lean muscles. They have a high metabolism, and it's hard for them to gain weight, including muscle and fat.

Mesomorphs – These people are naturally athletic with broad shoulders, slim waists and well-measured body fat. They gain muscle well and do well in many sports. They also gain and lose weight fairly easily.

Endomorphs – These people have large bone structure, are thicker around the waist and have a rounder shape with more body fat. They are naturally strong, but staying slim is more difficult for them.

Lifestyle habits can change the body type. Someone who was born an ectomorph (lean and slender with a fast metabolism) can morph his/her body into endomorph (round with more body fat) if sedentary activities and unhealthy eating habits persist. Alternatively, a person born an endomorph (round with more body fat) can change his/her body into mesomorph (athletic build) if physical activities and healthy eating habits persist.

What body type do you believe you closely resemble?

Food
Macronutrient Percentage

Since not all bodies were created the same, it stands to reason that we can't feed all bodies the same way, as well. Just like certain body types favor certain sports (e.g. ectomorphs usually excel in running), certain body types favor particular percentages of foods. All the distinctive body types on earth can't eat the same way and expect the same results, especially as we get older. Although every **macronutrient (macro)** is necessary—**proteins**, **carbohydrates** and **fats**—we can adjust the quantity of each macro that we consume to match our body type.

If our body is not an ectomorph (long and lean), we won't be able to eat as many carbohydrates as they do. And many people wouldn't do well with the high fat consumption that endomorphs may eat (good fats are our friends, not enemies). Once we know our body type, we will better understand how to best feed it in order to maintain a healthy weight. Although our **macro food percentage** may need to be tailored to fit our needs more specifically by a dietitian (especially if we have a long history of unhealthy eating and lack of exercise) there is a good rule of thumb for each body type. These macro percentages are recommended by the *International Sports Sciences Association.*

Out of their daily food consumption, **ectomorphs** should eat 25% protein, 55% carbohydrates and 20% fat.

Out of their daily food consumption, **mesomorphs** should eat 30% protein, 40% carbohydrates and 30% fat.

Out of their daily food consumption, **endomorphs** can eat 35% protein, 25% carbohydrates and 40% fats.

Once we know our macro food percentage, we can adjust the foods on our plate to match our body type. We want to take care, though, that the foods we choose from each macro are **nutritionally dense foods**. For example, the endomorph may not be able to eat the baked potato with his/her steak, but he/she can definitely get creamed spinach to go with it. And the ectomorph may not be able to eat the cheese on her/his salad, but she can have a whole-grain roll instead.

Rather than focusing on the foods we can't have, we need to focus on the abundance of foods we can have. We are so blessed with the variety of foods from which we can choose, and when we see how good the foods are on our own plate, we won't worry about what's on the plate of the person next to us.

What are your macronutrient percentages?

Faith
The Power of Self-control

*"But the Holy Spirit produces this kind of fruit in our lives: love, joy, peace, patience, kindness, goodness, faithfulness, gentleness, and **self-control**. There is no law against these things." (Galatians 5.22-23 NLT).*

The hand of God's favor and abundance is currently on America because we are a country founded on His principles in the Bible. This doesn't mean we are a perfect country with a perfect past, but our foundation was built on the solid Word of God and our influence has spread across the world. Though this foundation is currently shifting, we still enjoy the blessings of God's abundance. However, this bounty necessitates the Fruits of the Spirit, especially the last one listed in Galatians chapter five: **Self-control**.

When Jerusalem was destroyed by the Babylonians in 586 BC, the Jewish people in the Old Testament were taken to Babylon—**another richly blessed country at the time**. Daniel and his friends were selected to be trained to serve in King Nebuchadnezzar's court. They found themselves at the king's table, tempted by a great amount of **royal foods** that would defile them. They decided to go against the cultural expectations around them, and they ate to please the Lord. After only 10 days of abstaining from the royal foods, they proved to be healthier and fitter than all the others.

*"At the end of the ten days **they looked healthier and better nourished** than any of the young men who ate the royal food" (Daniel 1.15 NIV).*

We too find ourselves at the king's table every day in America. Though we are probably not called to the strict diet that Daniel and his friends had committed to, we do need to exert **self-control** when it comes to the amount, frequency and types of foods we choose to consume, especially if we have excess storage fat to lose. It will take effort at first because we have grown attached to our "royal eating," but after 10 days, we will feel such a difference in our entire existence that our new eating choices will be well worth it. And we will realize that the **King of the Universe** has already prepared us a table on earth that is chock-full of wonderfully tasting and nutritionally rich foods.

The principle is this: **We control food; food doesn't control us**. The Holy Spirit wants to guide us in our food consumption, and we can pray about every last bite we place on our lips. God won't condemn us, so there is no need to carry the burden of guilt, shame and worry. We simply need to wrestle into a higher level of intimacy and dependency on the Lord. God knows our struggle, and He will help us moment-to-moment and bite-to-bite. We simply need to ask the Holy Spirit to renew our minds, and give us His discerning palate of tasty food choices.

"Do not conform to the pattern of this world, but be transformed by the renewing of your mind. Then you

will be able to test and approve what God's will is--his good, pleasing and perfect will" (Romans 12.2 NIV).

Chapter 2

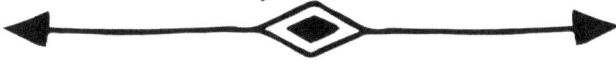

"But thanks be to God. He gives us the victory through our Lord Jesus Christ" (1 Corinthians 15.57 NIV).

Fitness
Exercise is Mandatory

All of us have different schedules, live in different environments and find ourselves in different seasons of life. When we are just starting our exercise routine, we should aim towards achieving **2.5 hours** of aerobic and/or anaerobic exercise a week. Once exercise becomes a normal part of our daily routine, we can work our way to achieving **5 hours** of physical activity a week.

We can wake up 30 minutes early for 5 days and walk our neighborhood. We can work out 30 minutes during lunch 5 days a week. We can do a 40-minute aerobic video 4 days a week after work. We can swing by the gym for 50 minutes 3 days a week. We can work out on an aerobic machine during our favorite shows every weeknight. And we can spend our weekends doing fun outdoor activities—going to the beach, playing a sport, hiking with our family, walking the malls, etc.

There are so many different ways to fit exercise into our schedules. As the old saying goes, **"Where there is a will, there is a way."** We all can look at our schedule and rearrange things to achieve the recommended hours of exercise. Sedentary activities are on a rise, so we need to be cognizant of adding physical activities into our day—even if it means wearing tennis shoes to work and doing lunges down the hallway during our coffee break or jump roping in a parking lot while our daughter does ballet or our son practices baseball.

Our body was designed to move, and our muscles will atrophy if they are not used on a regular basis. Because of the sedentary aspects of our current culture (cars, computers, cell phones, desk jobs, etc.), it is no longer a choice to exercise; **it is mandatory**. So we have to find the balance in our schedule that includes physical activity. We can start out slowly, working our way to being fitness pros.

Once we admit that exercise is an absolute must in our life, we will become creative with our time. We don't need a gym membership to get our daily exercise, though it wouldn't hurt. We can use the resources and environments around us. No matter who we are and where we find ourselves, we can start reaping a vast knowledge of exercise expertise that suits our daily needs. God wants us to take care of our "temples," so He will make a way when there doesn't seem to be a way. He will help us reorganize our schedule and get creative with our time, but we need to be open to new possibilities.

*"See, I am doing a new thing. Now it springs up; do you not perceive it? **I am making a way in the wilderness** and streams in the wasteland" (Isaiah 43.19 NIV).*

Our two main excuses not to exercise usually include **busyness** and **tiredness**. However, research shows that exercise actually fights **fatigue**, **depression**, **stress**, **anxiety**, **illness**, **injury** and **disease**. We can't afford not to exercise. The quality of our life on earth is at stake, so we need to take time to be proactive. If we are suffering from any of those negative hindrances in our life, we need to put on our running shoes and get moving. Surprisingly, though, we will soon find that once we integrate physical activities into our daily routine, we won't be able to imagine life without it. Our emotional, spiritual and physical well-being will skyrocket, and we won't want to lose the **amazing benefits that we reap from exercise**.

Food
Body Mass Index

Finding our **Body Mass Index** shows us how much of our body mass is made up of fat. Fat is not a bad thing. In fact, fat is one of our body's defense mechanism, preventing starvation and promoting health. Fat on our body is healthy within normal proportions. The problem occurs when we have too much or too little fat. Finding our Body Mass Index (BMI) will help determine whether we need to gain, lose or maintain weight. We may be a little apprehensive at first, but we must remember that awareness is the first key to winning the battle.

When calculating our BMI mathematically, we must remember that this number is a ballpark number. A mathematical formula does not account for gender, age or muscle mass. Also, children have their own BMI calculator. Advances in technology have given way to more accurate BMI calculating methods and machines that can be administered by health professionals, but for this book the mathematical BMI formula is useful as a starting point. We all have a fairly good idea if we need to lose, gain or maintain weight, but knowing our BMI gives our suspicions solid proof.

Body Mass Index

Fat percentage
Underweight = <18.5

Normal weight = 18.5–24.9
Overweight = 25–29.9
Obese = BMI of 30 or greater

Calculating Our BMI

Calculate BMI by dividing weight in pounds (lbs.) by height in inches (in) squared and multiplying by a conversion factor of 703.

This sounds pretty complicated, but it is easily performed with a calculator.

Example for a 140-pound person who is 5'7":

Weight = 140 lbs., Height = 5'7" (67")
Calculation: [140 ÷ (67)2] x 703 =

140/4,489 = .0312 x 703 = 21.92

22% BMI is within normal range.

People who have more lean body mass (muscle) because they lift weights will have higher BMI due to muscle hypertrophy. Also, endomorph body types will naturally have a higher BMI. There are numerous BMI calculators online that do the mathematical calculations for free. We must not become dismayed if we discover our BMI is not within normal range. We can start today making healthy choices that will promote our quality of life and physical health.

What is your Body Mass Index (BMI)?

Faith
The Power of Sowing

"Do not be deceived: God cannot be mocked. A man **reaps what he sows**. *Whoever sows to please their flesh, from the flesh will reap destruction; whoever sows to please the Spirit, from the Spirit will reap eternal life"* (Galatians 6.7-8 NIV).

No matter our body type, there is only one reason (other than genetics) why we find ourselves unhealthy and unhappy with our body: lifestyle choices. We must understand that if we are making unhealthy choices every day, we will reap an unhealthy life. There is no miracle cure to health and fitness. We must gain knowledge for healthy living and apply what we have learned.

Maybe we inherited unhealthy habits from our parents or maybe our own ignorance and/or compromise created unhealthy lifestyle behaviors. The enemy's desire for us to be flippant about our health is succeeding. Unhealthy living is the number one killer in the United States, leading to chronic diseases. We can no longer pretend that nothing is going on.

Just like Jesus, we each have a body and soul—and they are very much intertwined with each other. If we ignore the health of our body, every aspect of our person (mind, body, soul) will be affected. We can start today, reaping a harvest of health and fitness in our life by making simple changes. We may not be able to see the results right away, but we can have faith in God's promises that we will **"reap what we sow."** Our lifestyle changes won't be made in vain.

During those hard times when we want to give up and fall back into old patterns, we can tap into God's joy and peace and pour them into new, healthier patterns. God is the source of all that is good, and because we have the Holy Spirit inside of us, we have that Source available to us every moment of every day. When we get tired and want to give up and our endless sowing seems to reap only fields of fruitless emptiness, we have to remember that our hope is in the supernatural power of the Holy Spirit working in us, and He won't let us down. We will reap a harvest of health if we just keep going.

*"May the God of hope fill you with all **joy and peace as you trust in him**, so that you may overflow with hope by the **power of the Holy Spirit**" (Romans 15.13 NIV).*

Chapter 3

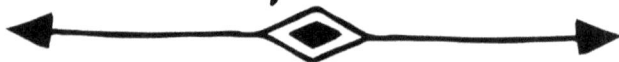

"I appeal to you therefore, brothers, by the mercies of God, to present your bodies as a living sacrifice, holy and acceptable to God, which is your spiritual worship" (Romans 12.1 ESV).

Fitness
Disuse vs. Age

Many people inaccurately believe that our lack of muscle strength is due to our age. Or they may think that as we age, our muscles become weaker. But that simply isn't the case. Age doesn't affect our muscles as much as **disuse does**. When we stop using our muscle strength, we will ultimately lose it. **We lose what we don't use**. Studies have shown that active individuals in their 60s have more muscle strength than sedentary individuals in their 30s. Age is no longer a viable excuse to why we have lost our strength.

As we age, our muscle disuse becomes more and more evident until we get to a point where we can't lift a kitchen appliance. The good news is that it is never too late to start an exercise program. We may not be able to jump right into bench presses and deadlifts, but we can begin to use the muscles that we have been ignoring. And we will discover that our body will come alive with every day we commit to exercising.

Astronauts in space can lose muscle strength in mere days, so we can't expect any less when we are doing sedentary activities every day. Some of these activities are necessary. Many of us work at a computer for hours a day, which is why we need to be aggressive about balancing our physical inactivity (driving, desk work, computer work, etc.) with physical activity (exercise, sports, outside hobbies, etc.). We have to look for relaxing hobbies that aren't sedentary and/or develop an exercise routine to move our body.

Seated television watching after a long day at the computer will only weaken us over the years. **And it's not fair to our body**, forcing it to watch active adults on TV while our own body wastes away. There is nothing particularly wrong with TV, **but if we give up our health for it, something needs to change**. We may need to choose a few of our favorite shows and cut the rest from our viewing, so we can refresh our bodies, minds and souls with gift of health. Or we can keep our body active—on an exercise machine or with body Calisthenics (exercises using body weight)— while watching TV. It may take a little discipline to train the body to move while the mind is engaged, but it can be done and our favorite shows won't be missed.

Remember where there is a will, there is a way. God will create streams in the desert. If we would only look around and stay open-minded, there will be endless possibilities to incorporate physical activity into our lifestyle. We don't have to turn our world upside-down to be healthy; we merely have to tilt it slightly. We have so many resources available to us that will help us to experience the power of a healthy lifestyle. We can listen to audiobooks while we walk the block. We can catch up on phone calls while we ride a stationary bike. We can engage in fun family time as we dance around the living room with our kids. We can enjoy a nice hike with family and friends. The options are endless.

Food
Macronutrients (Macros)

1 gram of **Protein** = 4 calories
1 gram of **Carbohydrate** = 4 calories
1 gram of **Fat** = 9 calories

Fad diets don't work for long because they lean heavily on consuming one macronutrient instead of implementing them all. **All three macros are important to a healthy diet.** We can tailor macros to fit what we want to eat according to our body type (ectomorph, mesomorph and endomorph). However, there are some foods that are higher quality than others. When we consume high calorie, low nutritional foods, we are literally starving our body of nutrients. We eat and eat, yet our body craves more because it is missing the necessary nutrients it needs to thrive.

The best way to loosen the grip of "comfort foods" is to inundate our diet with a variety of nutritionally packed, great tasting foods. That way our desire for "empty calories" won't be as strong. Instead of focusing on what we can't eat (unless we are having a "cheat meal," which we will discuss later), we can embrace all the amazing foods that God created for us. God provides us with a beautiful array of foods that can be divided into **three basic macronutrients (macros)** based on how they affect our body.

Proteins – They build and repair body tissues and structures. Proteins are made up of amino acids, which are the building blocks of our body. It is imperative to consume our protein macro percentage.

Carbohydrates (Carbs) – They are the main source of energy for our body, which include complex starchy carbs, complex fibrous carbs and simple carbs. Carb macros can be decreased when trying to lose weight and build muscle.

Fats – They are a high source of energy that helps signal fullness when we are eating. They aid our body in absorbing fat-soluble vitamins and provide fatty acids that cannot be sufficiently produced by the body. Fats eaten in proper proportion do not make us fat.

Each macro is necessary to our body's health within its required percent range. Too much of any one thing (other than God Himself) is never good. Water and oxygen are the two basic elements that we need to survive on earth, but give a body too much of each, and it will die. The same goes with food. We can't eat carbs all the time, ignoring necessary healthy fats and proteins, and expect our body to thrive without the building blocks of amino acids (vegetarians can receive complete proteins from non-animal products). Also, we can't eat only fats and proteins all the time, and expect our body to thrive without valuable fiber gained from carbs. We can integrate all three macros into our diets, knowing that we will be providing our body with all the nutrients it needs.

Faith
The Power of Today

"This is the day the LORD has made. We will rejoice and be glad in it" (Psalm 118.24 NLT).

Today is a very powerful day. It is the only day that we actually have the ability to make a difference and create changes. *Today* is the landscape for which the colors of our free will can move across the pages of our lives. We can learn from **yesterday**, but we can't change it. We can set goals for **tomorrow**, but we can't touch it. But **today** we can change and touch. Today is the day we can give our fitness, food and faith to the Lord, so He can guide us into a powerful new level of health in our life.

The only frustrating thing about *today* is that we rarely see the full picture created by our actions. It isn't until a bunch of days of action blend into the next that we can stand back and see what our efforts have displayed. Will we be pleased or shocked by the results? **Will our future-self be happy or dismayed by the choices we are making today?** We can keep that in mind that when we establish our *today*, so when we finally look up, we will be surrounded by the amazing fruits of our good choices.

When we begin to implement food and activity changes into our daily life, we won't experience the results right away. In fact, it may take months to finally feel and see the rewards of our new healthy lifestyle.

But rest assured, we will reap the benefits of healthy living. It's difficult to stick to the process of any transformation when we don't see results right away, but the harvest is being planted and it is only a matter of time before we reap the benefits of our efforts. We can focus on making wise choices today, knowing that our positive decisions will finally catch up with us.

Chapter 4

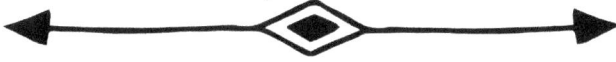

"So that you may not be sluggish, but imitators of those who through faith and patience inherit the promises" *(Hebrews 6.12 ESV).*

Fitness
Heart Health

The heart is the most important muscle in our body, and like all muscles, it needs exercise to be healthy. It may seem contradictory, but the harder we push our heart, the stronger our heart becomes (under normal circumstances). The stronger our heart becomes, the fewer times it has to beat to circulate the oxygen-rich blood from our lungs to the rest of our body. When we don't exercise, our heart becomes weaker, forcing it to beat more times per minute, per hour, per day and per lifetime.

When we routinely exercise, we can run down the street to catch a flyaway receipt without getting winded. We can reorganize the garage without having to take a break. We can walk up several flights of stairs without missing a beat. However, if we don't exercise, even the most simple of exercises, like getting out of bed, walking to the mailbox or even picking up a pet becomes tiresome. Our heart deserves better than that. If God has granted us a strong, healthy heart, we should embrace that gift.

The best way to discover the condition of our heart is to take our resting heart rate. We can lie down for several minutes, relaxing our body, and then use a timer to count how many beats our heart makes in 60 seconds by placing our index and middle fingers on our carotid artery located on the neck. Once we count how many times our heart has to beat in a minute, we will have a pretty good idea how strong our heart is. Anything over 80 beats per minute suggests that we are not exercising and our heart is weak. But this can all change. After 6 months of exercise, our resting heart rate can drop up to 10 beats per minute.

RESTING HEART RATE FOR WOMEN

Age	18-25	26-35	36-45	46-55	56-65	65+
Athlete	54-60	54-59	54-59	54-60	54-59	54-59
Excellent	61-65	60-64	60-64	61-65	60-64	60-64
Good	66-69	65-68	65-69	66-69	65-68	65-68
Above Average	70-73	69-72	70-73	70-73	69-73	69-72
Average	74-78	73-76	74-78	74-77	74-77	73-76
Below Average	79-84	77-82	79-84	78-83	78-83	77-84
Poor	85+	83+	85+	84+	84+	84+

RESTING HEART RATE FOR MEN

Age	18-25	26-35	36-45	46-55	56-65	65+
Athlete	49-55	49-54	50-56	50-57	51-56	50-55
Excellent	56-61	55-61	57-62	58-63	57-61	56-61
Good	62-65	62-65	63-66	64-67	62-67	62-65
Above Average	66-69	66-70	67-70	68-71	68-71	66-69
Average	70-73	71-74	71-75	72-76	72-75	70-73
Below Average	74-81	75-81	76-82	77-83	76-81	74-79
Poor	82+	82+	83+	84+	82+	80+

What is your resting heart rate?

Food
Basal Metabolic Rate (BMR)

Our metabolism is a combination of chemical reactions in our body that transfers the energy we consume to the energy we exert. Like fuel in a car, our metabolism takes the food we eat to provide energy for our body's inner functions and outer movements. This fuel is represented in a measurement called calories. **We consume calories when we eat. We exert calories when we exercise.**

1) A calorie is a measure of heat energy.
2) Food gives us energy when it is burned.
3) Fat is our storehouse of energy.
4) Food is fuel for our lives.

In order to correctly fuel our body type, we have to know how many calories our body needs every day. Once we know our basic caloric intake, we can adjust our food consumption, depending on whether we want to gain, lose or maintain our weight. Also, **knowing our Basal Metabolic Rate (the minimum calories our body needs to survive)** will help us not to overeat our calories, which causes us to gain several pounds every year.

Our Basal Metabolic Rate (BMR) is the calories (energy) we need to maintain our body's functions while awake at a rested state. This is our basic energy need and doesn't take into account our daily activity level. We can approximate our BMR with an easy formula, so we can monitor our food intake to ensure our actions create our desired result. Ignorance to how much we are eating is like trying to launch a rocket to the moon without analyzing the fuel necessary first. We must consider everything we put past our lips until healthy habits are formed, especially when we are trying to lose unwanted fat.

BMR Formula for Women:
BMR = 655 + (4.35 x weight in pounds) + (4.7 x height in inches) – (4.7 x age in years).

BMR Formula for Men:
BMR = 66 + (6.23 x weight in pounds) + (12.7 x height in inches) – (6.8 x age in year).

Example:
A 140-pound female who is 5'7" and 38 years old will have a BMR formula like this: 655 + 609 + 314.9 – 178.6 = 1,400.3 (calories a day). So this woman needs to eat at least 1,400 calories every day just to maintain her weight. If she has an active lifestyle, she will have to consume more calories to maintain weight or she will lose weight. If she eats several hundred calories above her BMR, she will gain a few pounds of body fat (stored energy) every year.

A simpler BMR formula is to multiply our weight by 10. So the 140-pound woman would need to eat 10x her body weight, which is again 1,400 calories. However, if we are trying to lose weight, we would multiply our **goal weight** (not our actual weight) by 10. For example, if a 160-pound woman wanted to lose 20 pounds, she would multiply her goal weight of 140 pounds by 10. She would require 1,400 calories a day (without exercise) to lose weight (instead of the 1,600 calories she would need to maintain her weight). If she implemented exercise into her diet, the calories burned would create an even larger caloric deficit, helping her to reach her goal weight even faster.

Therefore, the 160-pound woman would have a 200-calorie deficit in her diet each day if she switched from eating 1,600 calories to 1,400 calories. The woman might not be aware of it, but she may have been eating over her 1,600-calorie limit, which is causing her to gain weight steadily through the year. **There is approximately 3,500 calories in each pound of fat.** So depending on how many calories she eats above her BMR and activity level, she could gain a few pounds or several pounds over the long run. She'll want to make some adjustments, but with a little bit of time and effort, she can revolutionize her life.

What is your Basal Metabolic Rate (BMR)?

Faith
The Power of Positive Words

*"Let no corrupting talk come out of your mouths, but only such as **is good for building up**, as fits the occasion, that it may give grace to those who hear"* *(Ephesians 4.29 ESV).*

We live in the natural world, but our hearts have the imprint of a greater, spiritual world (Ecclesiastes 3.11). Eventually, heaven will be our home and eternity will be our reality. Right now our earthly home is encased, like a baby in a womb, in our spiritual home. The spiritual reality is greater than our natural reality because it is eternal. But until we make it home to heaven, we can open the power of heaven on earth with our words.

Since we have both flesh and spirit, we have the power to access both the natural and supernatural worlds. We have much power in our natural strengths and abilities to make a difference for the Kingdom of God, **but our truest strength is found in our words.** Our words have the power of life and death because they give us the ability to reach into the spiritual world and change our natural circumstances. We can use our words to claim the power of heaven to accomplish victory in our health today.

"Death and life are in the power of the tongue, and those who love it will eat its fruits" (Proverbs 18.21 ESV).

There is so much power in the spoken word. By our own mouths, we can speak a tree of life fruited with blessings (Proverbs 15.4). We can bless others (Proverbs 11.25). We can turn away wrath (Proverbs 15.1). We can bring health to our soul and body (Proverbs 16.24). We can even preserve our life (Proverbs 13.3). It's not a coincidence that Jesus is called the Word (John 1.1). He spoke salvation and redemption over creation by saying, "It is finished" on the cross (John 19.30). God used words to create all life, speaking everything into being. If God's words are that powerful, and we are made in His image, shouldn't we be wise about the words we choose to speak (Genesis 1.27)?

As we continue on our health experience, let's ensure that our words are speaking victory, blessing, abundance, strength, peace and power. Not only the words we speak, but the words we think and believe, as well. We can pave a path of success with our mouth. We must root out any negative beliefs, thoughts and words that try to attach themselves to our journey because they will sabotage our actions. We can claim the promises of God found in His Word to boldly walk into a new life of fitness and health. We can speak the 12 promises below every day and experience how the power of words radically changes our life.

- We are dressed in strength and our arms are strong. – Proverbs 31.17

- We can do all things through Christ who gives us strength. – Philippians 4.13
- God's power is strong in our weakness. – 2 Corinthians 12.9-10
- God will give us rest when we are weary. – Matthew 11.28-29
- God gives us power when we are weak and strength when we are powerless. – Isaiah 40.29-31
- We have the victory through Christ. – Romans 8.37-38
- Christ is giving us peace, so we don't have to be troubled or afraid. – John 14.27
- God's plans for us are for good, not disaster. – Jeremiah 29.11
- With God all things are possible. – Matthew 19.26
- The Lord is our strength and our helper. – Psalm 28.7
- God gives us a spirit of power, love and a sound mind. – 2 Timothy 1.7
- We can't possibly fathom the amazing things that God has prepared for us. – 1 Corinthians 2.9

Chapter 5

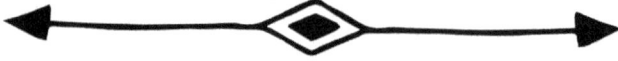

Fitness
Aerobic Exercise

There are two main types of exercise: **aerobic exercise** (cardio) and **anaerobic exercise** (strength training and high intensity training). In the most basic terms, **aerobic exercise allows the metabolism to use oxygen** to make chemical reactions to form energy. And **anaerobic exercise makes the metabolism use chemical reactions without oxygen** to form energy. Both types of exercise will strengthen the body and decrease the resting heart rate, but they do achieve varying results.

Aerobic exercise is great for beginners, since engaging in most anaerobic activities (sports, bodybuilding, jumping rope, sprints, etc.) requires a foundation of aerobic strength first. Aerobic exercise forces the heart to keep up with the oxygen demands placed on the body to produce the energy needed for consistent, moderate movements. It also elevates our metabolism, helping us to burn more calories. Our heart gets stronger as it pushes our metabolism to supply the oxygen demands on the body during aerobic exercise.

Our main goal when performing aerobic exercise is to meet our **target heart rate** for the middle portion of our work out—the time between our **warm up** and **cool down**. When just starting out, we may not be able to keep this target heart rate for more than 20 minutes (with a five minute warm up and five minute cool down), but as we continue, each week we should be able to add 5 minutes to our work out time. Once we reach our goal of 40 minutes, we can begin to increase the intensity of our exercise and maintain a higher target heart rate.

Most aerobic machines have a heart rate monitor located somewhere near the handlebars. If a heart rate monitor is not present, we can check our own heart rate to ensure we are hitting our target. We do this by using the same method that we used to find our resting heart rate. We place our middle finger and index fingers on our carotid artery located on our neck. However, this time we only count the beats that occur in 10 seconds, and we can multiply that number by 6 to estimate our **beats per minute**. We can also buy a personal heart rate monitor that we wear on our body.

Unless we want to know our exact number, though, as long as we are moderately uncomfortable during the middle portion of our work out, we should be hitting our target heart rate. For example, if we are trying to keep a conversation while exercising, it should be obvious to the listener that we are working out. If we are conversing without having to catch our breath while working out, we may need to increase the intensity.

We can find our target heart rate (HR) that corresponds with our age, located in the middle column of the following table. When we begin our work out routine (**remember we want to exercise 2.5 hours a week, working our way to 5 hours a week**), we can commit to 30 minutes 5 days a week, 40 minutes 4 days a week or 50 minutes 3 days a week. We can use the same exercise work out in the beginning (stationary bike, walking, stair climbing, swimming, etc.), but when our heart and body get proficient at a certain exercise, we will want to add a variety of other aerobic exercises to our routine and increase the intensity as our heart gets stronger. Otherwise, our aerobic strength will stagnate. Once our aerobic foundation becomes strong, we can also start incorporating a few anaerobic exercises into our routine, as well.

Target Heart Rate in Beats Per Minute

Age	Target HR 50-85%	Maximum HR 100%
20	100-170	200
30	95-162	190
35	93-157	185
40	90-153	180
45	88-149	175
50	85-145	170
55	83-140	165
60	80-136	160
65	78-132	155
70	75-128	150

The right column of the table shows **maximum heart rate**. Any heart rate hitting over 85% or more places us outside of aerobic activity and into anaerobic activity. Anaerobic activity cannot last for more than **2 minutes** or until our muscles fatigue and we need to stop to regain our strength. We will discuss anaerobic exercise in the following chapter.

Food
Creating Calorie Deficit

Once we find our average caloric needs from our BMR, we can now decide how many calories we need to consume in order to reach our goal. This will help us fuel our body more effectively, and we can manipulate our calories to gain, lose or maintain weight. Let's take the woman who weighs 160 pounds.

She wants to lose 20 pounds. If each pound of fat has 3,500 calories, she would have to burn approximately 70,000 calories to lose 20 pounds (3,500 x 20). When we divide the total calories that she needs to burn (70,000 calories in all) by the 200 calorie deficit the woman has committed to (eating 1,400 calories instead of 1,600 calories a day), we find that it will take her approximately 350 days to lose 20 pounds, which is about a year.

This may seem like an eternity, but we want lasting change—not the ups and downs of losing and gaining weight. We need to focus on transforming an unhealthy lifestyle into a healthy lifestyle that lasts a lifetime. Quick fixes just don't work. We don't simply want to change our body; we want to change our overall health. Skinny people can be just as unhealthy as overweight people, so we want to focus on making results that count.

When caloric intake exceeds caloric output, the extra carbs, protein and fats are stored as fat in the body. The body stores fat in order to prepare for future famines. Those of us living in America are not foreseeing any famine hitting soon, so if our BMI is in the overweight or obese range, we will have to create our own "famine" to lose the extra weight. But we don't have to worry: this famine won't cause us to starve from hunger. It will merely cause us to lose the weight that is holding us back.

There are about 3,500 calories in every pound of fat. Therefore, if we would like to lose a pound a week, we must have a 500-calorie deficit every day (500 x 7 = 3,500). However, we should not go under 1,200 calories in a day because our metabolism will slow down in preparation of the worst—starving. When our metabolism slows, we will burn fewer calories and now we've just sabotaged our weight loss goals.

The best way to lose weight is to have a 250-calorie deficit from our BMR in order to lose 1 pound every two weeks (250 x 14 = 3,500). This will ensure that our metabolism doesn't go into "self-preservation mode" by slowing down. Moreover, a 250-deficit each day won't hinder our lifestyle too much. With proper planning, we can still go out to eat with friends and eat the same meals as our family. A 250-deficit is really just a candy bar, bag of chips or sugary latte that we don't need to consume anyway. Once we learn to embrace the low calorie, high nutritional foods that God has given us, the 250 calories won't be missed.

When we are in a calorie deficit, our body may feel hungry and send out "starving signals," but rest assured we are not starving. In fact, we are still probably eating better than much of the world. Our body doesn't know the difference between dieting and starving, so we will have to wield some self-control to beat our urges. However, 250-calorie deficit will help us not feel too hungry, and we can control our hunger, knowing that our next meal is just around the corner.

Losing weight: We must burn more calories than we consume.

Gaining weight: We must burn fewer calories than we consume.

Maintaining weight: We must burn the same calories that we consume.

What is your daily caloric intake goal?

Faith
The Power of Maintaining

"Jesus answered, 'How can the guests of the bridegroom fast while he is with them? They cannot, so long as they have him with them. But the time will come when the bridegroom will be taken from them, and on that day they will fast'" (Mark 2.19-20 NIV).

It is interesting how much control we can really have over our body when we put our mind and will to it. We actually have the ability to gain, lose and maintain weight, and we don't need a miracle pill to help us. God designed the body with amazing transformational ability, and He's given us full reign to create our body into any image we desire. So why do we struggle so much to change our body? We struggle with not being able to move our weight according to our desire for two reasons: **knowledge and self-control**.

Obtaining fitness and nutritional knowledge is easy if we make time to do it. Just like anything in life, there is an element of science and logic to managing our body and health. Even in a relationship (a more abstract concept) the basic truth is that if we work at it, the relationship will thrive makes sense (assuming both people are doing their part). We can't completely ignore a relationship and expect it to do well. The same is true for our body. **We can't completely ignore our body and expect it to do well.** Once we gain the physical and nutritional information we need, managing our weight should be doable and the sacrifices required will make sense because we better understand the process.

It's been stated before, **but wielding self-control is difficult since we live in a prosperous and blessed nation like America**. God designed our body with the feast and famine principle in mind. During the Bible times, **the people would experience times of feasting and times of famine regularly**. A drought would hit, and the people would not have enough food to eat. But then the crops would come in, and God commanded His people to feast. The rest of the time, people would maintain their weight—food was eaten to give people the necessary energy they needed to achieve their daily activities.

God calls all His children to times when they **fast** (assert self-control over their food intake) **and feast** (celebrate God's blessings by eating richly), and the rest of the time we simply **maintain**. The problem today is we do too much feasting and not enough fasting. We eat like kings every day and forget what Proverbs says about eating too much from the king's table.

"When you sit to dine with a ruler, note well what is before you, and put a knife to your throat if you are given to gluttony" (Proverbs 23.1-2 NIV).

Jesus told His disciples that *"...everyone who has been given much, much will be demanded; and from the one who has been entrusted with much, much more will be asked" (Luke 12.48 NIV).* What does this mean for us living in a prosperous nation? We have God's hand of blessing on us. As of now, we have an abundance of the "king's food" at our disposal. The burden of that blessing is that we need to obediently choose to walk in "fasting" situations when we feel the weight of our "feasting" creeping over us—literally. This doesn't mean we have to fast all foods (unless we are fasting for spiritual reasons), but it does mean we can fast the amount of food we eat and the types of food we eat. **Creating a 250-calorie deficit is a type of self-implemented fast**. And once we lose our feasting weight, we can go back to simply maintaining.

We all have a "sweet spot" in our weight that makes us feel good and look great. However, it is always best to allow for a minimum 5-pound fluctuation range. Our body weight will go up and down a few pounds for various biological, cultural and environmental reasons, and we can't get bent out of shape if the scale reads a 2-pound increase. If our clothes are fitting fine and we know we've been keeping up with our exercise and eating routine, there's no reason to even step on a scale.

"For the Spirit God gave us does not make us timid, but gives us power, love and self-discipline" (2 Timothy 1.7 NIV).

Chapter 6

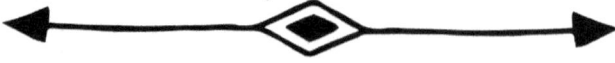

"Commit everything you do to the Lord. Trust him, and he will help you" (Psalm 37.5 NLT).

Fitness
Anaerobic Exercise

Anaerobic exercise does not use oxygen. This means when we do anaerobic exercise, our metabolism has to use chemical reactions to produce energy without oxygen. The intensity of the anaerobic exercise is so great that our heart can't keep up with the oxygen demands. Unlike aerobic exercise, we can't maintain the anaerobic intensity for more than 2 minutes before our muscles fatigue.

For this reason, anaerobic exercise is always done in sets of short intervals. When we engage in the anaerobic exercise of **strength or resistance training**, we are actually tearing our muscle fibers by forcing them to contract against the heavy weight. Only when we tear muscles will they become stronger. The heavier we lift, the less time we can hold the weight, and the more time we will have to rest afterward. If we are lifting weights to our max, we will have to rest after every set.

Moreover, during anaerobic exercise, we are getting our heart rate up to its max (85% or more), which is why we need a solid foundation of aerobic strength before we start an anaerobic workout routine. When we are engaging in the anaerobic exercise of **High Intensity Interval Training (HIIT)**, we want to push our heart rate to its max in short, intense bursts that can't be maintained for very long (around 20-60 seconds). We can use almost any aerobic exercise and turn it into an anaerobic exercise if we push our body and heart rate to the max. The chemical reactions that make the energy for anaerobic exercise creates a substance called **lactic acid**.

Most of the lactic acid in the muscles goes to the liver to be processed; however, some of it stays in the muscles, causing fatigue and soreness. To help reduce the effects of lactic acid build up we can drink lots of water, make sure we warm up and cool down, incorporate stretching and eat nutritionally dense foods packed with vitamins and minerals.

After anaerobic exercise is complete, there exists an oxygen debt in the body, which causes the heart rate to stay elevated and keeps the metabolism burning calories to replenish the oxygen levels. This heightened metabolism and heart rate can last for several minutes up to several hours after the exercise is complete, depending on the intensity of the workout. For this reason, many people prefer to do short, intense bursts of anaerobic exercise in order to boost their metabolism with great effectiveness in a shorter amount of time.

Age	Target HR 50-85%	Maximum HR 100%
20	100-170	200
30	95-162	190
35	93-157	185
40	90-153	180
45	88-149	175
50	85-145	170
55	83-140	165
60	80-136	160
65	78-132	155
70	75-128	150

In the right column is our maximum heart rate. Like stated earlier, if our heart rate is already high because our heart is weak (due to the lack of exercise), it won't take much to hit our max heart rate. And when we hit it, we won't stay there for very long because our muscles will fatigue, and they will tear if we are strength training. However, once we've committed to an aerobic routine for several months and our heart becomes stronger, we will want to implement more anaerobic exercises into our workout routine. Many people have their own routine based on the results they want to achieve (**especially if they are in competitive sports**), but for the rest of us a good rule of thumb is to do **three days of aerobic exercises a week and two days of anaerobic exercises a week**.

Food
Macro Breakdown

The woman from our previous example weighs 160 pounds, but she wants to weight 140 pounds. She will have to lose 20 pounds and achieve a 70,000-calorie deficit (200-calorie a day) over one year. She is going to consume 1,400 calories every day to reach her goal. Now we have to decide her body type and divide her daily caloric intake by the percentage for each macro she will consume.

Ectomorphs = 25% proteins, 55% carbohydrates and 20% fats.

Mesomorphs = 30% proteins, 40% carbohydrates and 30% fats.

Endomorphs = 35% proteins, 25% carbohydrates and 40% fats.

Let's assume that she has an endomorph body type. She will want to eat **35% protein**, **25% carbs** and **40% fats**. We can do the math by dividing her total daily caloric intake by each percentage.

Example:
1,400 (BMR) x .35 (percent of proteins) = **490 calories of proteins**

1,400 (BMR) x .25 (percent of carbs) = **350 calories of carbs**

45

1,400 (BMR) x .40 (percent of fats) = **560 calories of fats**

Now we can convert those calories into grams (g), which is how foods are quantified on nutritional labels located on the packaging of each item.

1 gram of Protein = **4 calories**
1 gram of Carbohydrate = **4 calories**
1 gram of Fat = **9 calories**

- Protein in calories (490) / 4 (calories per gram) = **122.5 grams of proteins** per day.

- Carbs in calories (350) / 4 (calories per gram) = **87.5 grams of carbs** per day.

- Fat in calories (560) / 9 (calories per gram)   = **62.2 grams of fats** per day.

Again, this will be hard for us to calculate for our daily food consumption without a calorie counter app. We live in a new culture that is changing every day. We have different temptations and struggles than people did 50 years ago. We have unhealthy foods all around us 24/7, so we need help while we learn to make healthy choices. Once our healthy habits are in place, we don't have to rely so heavily on technology to guide us. Until then, however, we need to use every resource at our disposal.

Moreover, many health professionals suggest adjusting our macros for a short time to kick-start our weight loss. This macro breakdown should only be done for a short period of time in order to accelerate our weight loss. While losing weight and/or gaining muscle, it is recommended to have the following macro percentages: **40% proteins, 20% carbs and 40% fats**. However, these percentages should not be maintained for prolonged periods of time. Once we lose our desired "kick-start" weight, we can return our macro intake back to the recommended percentages for our body type.

Example:
1,400 (BMR) x .4 (proteins) = 560
1,400 (BMR) x .2 (carbs) = 280
1,400 (BMR) x .4 (fats) = 560

Convert to Grams for Macros

- Proteins in calories (560) / 4 (calories per gram) = **140 grams** of carbs per day

- Carbs in calories (280) / 4 (calories per gram) = **70 grams** of carbs per day

- Fats in calories (560) / 9 (calories per gram) = **62.2 grams** of protein per day

Please note that if we are going to create a calorie deficit in order to burn excess fat storage, we will have to be more precise with the foods we choose to eat. We want to ensure that we consume all the necessary vitamins and minerals that our body needs to be healthy. Taking a multivitamin every day will make sure we are not lacking any of our necessary nutrients. However, if we are eating a minimum of five servings of colorful fruits and vegetables a day, we should be getting almost everything that our body needs.

Faith
The Power of Macros

"Taste and see that the LORD is good; blessed is the one who takes refuge in him" (Psalm 34.8 NIV).

There are three things that the body needs: **Carbohydrates (Carbs), Proteins and Fats**. These are called macronutrient (macros) because they are the three foundational nutrients of the body. Some fad diets will tell us to avoid one macro or to only eat another macro, but in most situations this is not healthy or balanced.

Each macro fulfills a specially designed purpose in the body. Carbs are the main source of energy to the body. Proteins provide amino acids, the basic building block of the body. And Fats (healthy fats) have many necessary benefits, including protecting the body's organs, absorbing vitamins, creating hormones, etc. We need all three macros in order to have a nutritionally integrated diet. Plus, each macro brings its own flavors and textures to our palates, and they work together to make our eating experience much more enjoyable.

The problem occurs in our diets when we eat our macronutrients out of balance, such as too many carbs and not enough protein or when we eat processed substitutes of healthy macros, such as trans fats and processed sugars and carbs instead of good fats and complex carbs.

Balance and authenticity are the keys to enjoying foods that keep us energized, healthy and looking and feeling great. We can run this same theme of **balance and authenticity** into our spiritual lives. We have three fundamental macronutrients to a healthy soul—**prayer and worship, Bible reading and meditation and fellowship and service**. All three of these macro spiritual nutrients are necessary for us to achieve a healthy spiritual life for the Lord.

First, **we can compare our prayer and worship to carbohydrates**. Carbs give our body energy and help us to achieve all our activities for the day. They are easy to absorb and instantly make us feel good. Just like carbs, prayer and worship maintain our spiritual activity and give us a boost of energy when we are running low. Prayer and worship is something we must be doing all throughout our day if we are going to victoriously achieve the goals that God has set for us. They keep our heavenly momentum going and prevent us from falling into defeat and despair.

"Jesus answered, 'It is written: 'Man shall not live on bread alone, but on every word that comes from the mouth of God'" (Matthew 4.4 NIV).

Next, **we can compare our Bible reading and meditation to proteins**. Just like protein provides us the basic elements (amino acids) to build our muscle, Bible reading and meditation provide us the basic elements (truth and revelation) to grow our spiritual muscles. In order to grow muscle, we must break it first. However, if we are not consuming enough protein, instead of rebuilding muscle, our muscle will deteriorate. The same goes for our spiritual lives.

God breaks us in order to build us up stronger in Him, but if we are not "eating" from His Word, we can't fully rebuild our spiritual muscles back up. **Instead of growing stronger in Christ, we will become bitter and spiritually weaker.** But if we consume God's Word by reading the Bible, the breaking will only lead to stronger faith. The Bible is the prime source of our protein, **like our ultimate complete protein**. But we can also consume of mix of God's Word through literature, music, movies, sermons, etc., which are like **incomplete proteins**, combining together to form a greater revelation of the Bible.

"When your words came, I ate them; they were my joy and my heart's delight, for I bear your name, LORD God Almighty" (Jeremiah 15.16 NIV).

Last, **we can compare fellowship and service to fats.** Healthy fats offer the body many necessary benefits, but their main role is to protect our body with energy stores in case of a famine. The same goes for our spiritual lives. Godly fellowship lines our spiritual lives with much needed "cushion," especially when we feel like we are spiritually starving. Sometimes a simple word of encouragement or a nod of understanding from someone helps us get through a particularly difficult time in our lives. We can borrow sustenance from others when we find ourselves in a season of a spiritual deficit.

Moreover, godly service is our way of giving from our abundance (stored fats) to others who are spiritually starving. We can serve others from the overflow of what God has already given us. Not only are we blessing them with much needed "soul nutrients," but we are honoring God with the talents and abilities that He has placed within us. This form of service is God's highest plan for us. He wants us to love Him and love others as ourselves, which implies that we must love ourselves and treat our body, mind and soul with love, respect and understanding, so we can adequately love, respect and understand others. When we fully submit to God and His Spirit, He will ensure that our spiritual macros are balanced and authentic, so we can be a good source of nutrition and substance to others.

"Therefore encourage one another and build each other up, just as in fact you are doing" (1 Thessalonians 5.11 NIV).

Chapter 7

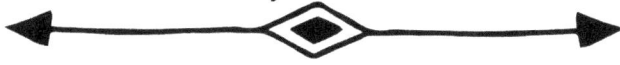

"I discipline my body like an athlete, training it to do what it should. Otherwise, I fear that after preaching to others I myself might be disqualified" (1 Corinthians 9.27 NLT).

Fitness
Aerobic Saturation and Calories

Getting our heart rate up for a lengthy period of time not only strengthens our heart and boosts our metabolism; it also forces us to keep a sustained elevation of oxygen saturation, which strengthens our cardiopulmonary system that supplies nutrients to our entire body, including our muscles. During aerobic exercise, our heart and lungs become stronger and more efficient, and our blood vessels grow in number and size.

Since blood vessels are important for carrying nutrients and oxygen to our muscles and carrying waste away, it stands to reason that aerobic exercise is important for muscle growth during anaerobic strength training—carrying away waste during muscle breakdown and bringing nutrients during rebuilding. For this reason, many people place importance on both aerobic and anaerobic exercise for achieving stellar health.

Below is a list of aerobic exercises and average calories they each burn per hour. The calorie counter app that we have downloaded will also have a working list of aerobic exercises and their calories burned. On the days we exercise, we can minus the burned calories from that day's total calorie intake, which means we can eat more nutritionally dense foods to fuel our body. Boosting our metabolism to burn more calories should not be our only focus while doing aerobic exercise. We want to ensure that we hit our target heart rate, so we can strengthen our heart. And we want to flood our body with oxygen, strengthening our cardiopulmonary system.

Aerobic Exercise	Calories Burned
Aerobics, general	380-605
Calisthenics, light	207-326
Cycling, moderate	472-745
Hiking, moderate	354-558
Rowing Machine, moderate	413-651
Running, moderate	472-745
Ski Machine	413-651
Stair Machine	531-838
Stationary Bike, moderate	413-651
Swimming, moderate	413-651
Walking, moderate	195-307

Research has shown that aerobic exercise increases energy, improves sleep, diminishes chemicals caused by stress and anxiety, encourages relaxation, improves mental awareness, reduces depression, fights heart disease, prevents injury, and burns unwanted fat stores. The benefits of aerobic exercise go beyond our physical well-being by promoting mental and emotional health, as well. Our entire quality of life is transformed when we take time to move our body. It's time to consider exercise a mandatory part of our day.

Food
Total Daily Energy Expenditure

If we happen to be engaged in a very active lifestyle, we can add slightly more calories to our daily caloric intake. We can adjust our BMR to our **Total Daily Energy Expenditure (TDEE).** This formula is for those of us who have careers and/or pastimes that engage us in daily activity (park ranger, childcare provider, construction worker, grounds keeper, surfer, etc.). However, if we are trying to lose weight, and our activity level is sedentary, it's best just to stick with our BMR number. If we are simply **maintaining weight**, though, it would be good to account for our activity level and adjust our calories to ensure that our body is properly fueled. Otherwise, we can add our calories burned during exercise to our calorie counter on the days we work out.

Our BMR (Basal Metabolic Rate) plus our Activity Level = our Total Daily Energy Expenditure (TDEE).

Sedentary	1.2-1.3
Lightly active	**1.4-1.5**
Active	**1.6-1.7**
Very active	**1.8-2.0**

If the woman from our example who weighs 160 pounds reaches her goal weight of 140 pounds, she will want to adjust her caloric intake to her **TDEE** in order to maintain her weight. She will multiply her BMR of 1,400 calories according to her lifestyle. If she works at a desk job, she will calculate her BMR to the sedentary category.

Example:
1,400 (BMR) x 1.2 (Sedentary) = 1,680 calories she can consume every day.

If she engages in an exercise activity, she can add those calories burned to her total caloric intake for that day. For example, if she walks the treadmill for 30 minutes at a moderate speed, she can add approximately 200 calories to her TDEE: **1,680 + 200 = 1,880 calories.** This will seem like a lot of available calories to her, especially after a year of cutting calories to lose excess weight. But when we are maintaining weight, we can enjoy a higher caloric intake each day, particularly when we exercise.

When we finally get to a point that we only have to maintain weight, we simply need to make sure that each day we have an equal energy balance: the energy we consume in foods matches the energy we exert with our BMR and activity level. The main reason we have to closely monitor this balance is because our homes, schools, jobs, communities and cities are flooded with foods. There seems to be a holiday every month and other reasons to celebrate sprinkled in between—birthdays, retirement parties, graduations, weekends, etc. We can jump from feast to feast, consuming empty party foods and desserts, and before we know it, we now have to lose weight again. We have to be proactive by planning our calories to adjust for celebrations, by eating smaller portions of party foods and desserts, by offering healthier foods when hosting or by simply saying, "No thank you."

What is your Total Daily Energy Expenditure (TDEE)?

Faith
The Power of Obedience

Obedience is a subject that is greatly misunderstood and devalued in our society, but its importance to our walk of faith is no less essential today. **If we don't learn obedience, we will completely miss out on the best life that God has for us.** Individuals can have talent, knowledge and charisma, but without the fortified roots of obedience, their intentions will be empty of action and the their lives will be void of results. **Obedience is the energy force that keeps us going even when everything inside of us tells us to quit.**

The key to an elevated life with Christ is obedience—it lifts us up out of our selfish path of mediocrity and sets us on glorious wings of God (Isaiah 40.31). On our own, we may try to avoid suffering through the hardships necessary to establish the fullness of God's glory in our lives. But it is out of the struggle that God's glory shines brightest, and only obedience will keep our resolve strong and our diligence unyielding to continue even when our path gets hard. Our obedience can be buffered by hope and protected by faith, but when the slightest ray of beauty can't be seen in our circumstances, obedience will maintain the steadfastness of our course.

"Yet what we suffer now is nothing compared to the glory he will reveal to us later" (Romans 8.18 NLT).

The truth of obedience is seen in the crucifixion of our Lord, Jesus Christ. He was about to experience sin and separation from His Father, and He asked God to "please take this cup of suffering away from me." But out of a heart of obedience, Jesus added the final words: **"Yet I want your will to be done, not mine"** (Luke 22.42 NLT). This awesome act of obedience even unto a physical and spiritual death to take the sins of the world unleashed the greatest demonstration of God's glory onto the earth— **salvation from sin and victory over death.**

We can learn from Jesus' example. If we know that God is asking us to shed, gain or maintain weight in order to get our health under control, we must be obedient to the steps necessary to achieve this victory. To be sure, the enemy will come out against us in full force when we resolve to transform our lifestyle for Christ. We will experience attacks emotionally, physically and spiritually and the storms of this world will seem to pound against us, willing us to give up our health journey. But keep the courage and stay strong. God has a glory He is just waiting to unleash in our lives, but we need to continue taking those obedient steps that are transforming our life.

"Have I not commanded you? Be strong and courageous. Do not be afraid; do not be discouraged, for the LORD your God will be with you wherever you go" (Joshua 1.9 NIV).

Chapter 8

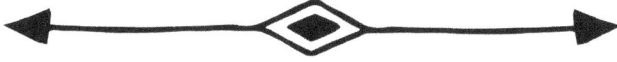

"Work willingly at whatever you do, as though you were working for the Lord rather than for people" *(Colossians 3.23 NLT).*

Fitness
High Intensity Interval Training (HIIT)

Once our aerobic stamina is strong, we can begin to dabble in a little High Intensity Interval Training (HIIT). Kids do HIIT all the time when they play, and it is usually during this intense playtime that parents say, "Calm down. Someone is going to get hurt." HIIT is when we achieve our max heart rate of 85% or more. When we watch kids reach this point, they can't maintain it for long (no more than 2 minutes if they have reached their max). They usually have to sit down after a moment and catch their breath until they feel able to set out again. The human body was created to achieve its max heart rate every once in a while. However, our lifestyle today does not offer many reasons to get to this point. That's why we have to seek those moments out.

One very important aspect of HIIT is ensuring that our form is correct. Many times when we are going all out and our heart is pumping at its max, we tend to become oblivious to the proper procedure for the exercise we are doing. We are so focused on getting the intense moment over with that our movements stray from protocol. That's why we need to take special care when doing High Intensity Interval Training work out videos, sprints, cardio machines and calisthenics. We don't want to injure our body. For example, when we are trying to do as many push-ups as possible in twenty seconds, we are going so fast that our form may get sloppy. We can injure our shoulders doing quick, incorrect push-ups, and we may not realize it until the next day when our shoulders ache.

The best way to avoid injury is to practice each exercise move slowly, making sure that our form is correct before we even begin. We can also do the exercise moves in front of a mirror if the form allows. Also, we can have people watch us while we do the exercise, so they can monitor our movements. Exercise is supposed to prevent injury by making every single facet of our body stronger, so we don't want to sabotage our body by using incorrect form. The goal for exercise is to prevent injury, not cause injury. So we must stay safe and keep good form.

A HIIT workout routine can be done for 20 minutes – 40 minutes, though many people believe that more than 30 minutes is too much. The reason why it's called "interval training" is because it is "high intensity," meaning we will go to failure during the intense parts and rest during the intervals. We can make almost any aerobic exercise into a HIIT work out, as long as we are hitting our max heart rate. A good HIIT work out to begin with is sprints. When we first start an aerobic exercise like walking, we may be only able to maintain 20 minutes of cardio with 5 minute cool down and warm up. Every week we want to add 5 minutes to our walk time. Once we hit 40 minutes of nonstop aerobic walking, we can begin to increase the intensity. We go from light walking to speed walking to light jogging to moderate jogging. Once a 40-minute jog becomes a piece of cake for us, we can begin HIIT sprints. This will ensure that our weight loss and fitness strength do not plateau.

There are many ways to divide our time during a HIIT routine, but the basic rule is to do 20-60 seconds high intensity, making sure our body switches from aerobic (with oxygen) to anaerobic (without oxygen) and that we go from our target heart rate to our max heart rate. So with our sprints, we want to make sure we get a 5-minute warm up, waking our muscles up and getting them ready for the work out. Once our body is warmed up, we can start our first high intensity sprint. We can start out with 20 seconds, running (with good form) as fast as we possibly can. Then we slow to a walk to allow our heart rate to come back down.

The time for rest is debated, but it's best to rest until we feel ready to sprint again (at least double the time we maintained our max heart rate). So if we sprinted for 20 seconds, we should rest for at least 40 seconds or more until we are ready to hit our max heart rate again. After we do our 25 minutes of HIIT, we will be exhausted but feeling great. Our hearts, lungs, muscles have been worked. Our metabolism has been boosted and will continue to stay elevated throughout the day. Our mood is lifted. We are feeling great. And we only had to sacrifice 25 minutes of our day.

We can do HIIT on almost any cardio machine at the gym—row machine, stair machine, stationary bike, elliptical and/or treadmill. We can also use calisthenics—work out moves using our own body weight. Doing HIIT with calisthenics is a great way to get a full body work out at home, on vacation or on a business trip. We can do intervals of sit-ups, squats, push-ups, dips, mountain climbers, burpees, lunges, jumping jacks and more. All we have to do is pick out a handful of exercises and do each one with rest intervals in between. We can do several sets of our chosen exercises until we reach our desired work out time. The great thing about using HIIT with calisthenics is that there is no equipment necessary, unless we want to throw in a jump rope, pull-up bar and/or step-up box. Just imagine it: a full body work out done before the kids wake up, during our lunch break, during our favorite night time show or right before bed. There's no excuse not to get into great shape.

Food
Proteins

There are three macros in the human diet that we have already discussed: **proteins**, **carbohydrates** and **fats**. Every body type (ectomorph, mesomorph and endomorph) should consume foods from all three macronutrients every day in their designated percentages. Proteins are especially important if we want to build greater muscle mass, which is muscle hypertrophy. Most bodybuilders will add protein supplements (protein drinks and bars) to their diets every day to ensure they consume their protein percentage. Having protein with every meal will encourage us to feel full and prevent us from overeating.

Proteins are made up of amino acids, which are the building blocks of our cells. If a food gives us all the essential amino acids we need, it is called a **complete protein**. If a food gives us only some of the essential amino acids we need, it is called an **incomplete protein**. We should consume complete proteins with every meal, which can include a combination of incomplete proteins to form a complete protein. These incomplete protein food combinations have been prevalent on plates for generations, which is why peanut butter on bread and rice and beans are notorious meal options.

Animal complete proteins include eggs, dairy, fish, poultry, red meat, game meat and pork.

Plant complete proteins include quinoa, flaxseed, amaranth, soybeans, buckwheat, hempseed and chia.

Combined incomplete proteins include grains and legumes (**rice and beans**), nuts/seeds and legumes (**hummus**) and nuts/seeds and grains (**peanut butter on whole wheat bread**).

The combined incomplete proteins contain much more carbohydrates than animal proteins, which will need to be considered when we calculate our daily consumption percentage of each macro for our body type. Endomorphs may find it difficult to eat their percentage of protein without going over their percentage of carbs on a strictly vegetarian diet. Vegetarians should rely on the complete protein plant foods and combinations of the incomplete protein plant foods for every meal in order to adequately consume their protein percentage and to stay full.

Also, the serving size restaurants offer us can be double or even triple the standard protein serving size. A serving size is usually the size of the palm of our hand, so we need to be careful to order smaller portions when dining out. Moreover, eating a variety of proteins is healthier than eating too much of one type of protein source. We may be tempted to overeat red meat—steak, hamburgers, ribs, brisket, pot roast, etc.—but we need to ensure that we are balancing our protein intake with fish, turkey, chicken, lean pork, game meat, etc. Each diverse protein adds unique nutritional value to our body.

Eggs are also excellent sources of protein; however, the fat in the egg yolk can add up, making us go over in our fat percentage. A good idea when making scrambled eggs is to add equal portions of eggs to egg whites (egg whites can be purchased in separate cartons for easy use). This way we get plenty of protein without going over in fat. Finally, we want to limit our intake of processed meats, like sausage, lunchmeat, bacon, salami and hot dogs. They are extremely high in sodium and other preservatives that our body will eventually have to process and flush out. When looking at processed meats, it's best to choose the ones with low sodium, low saturated fats and no nitrates.

Faith
The Power of Good Form

Good form saves us energy, prevents injury and builds muscles effectively because we are performing our routine properly. It is imperative when starting a strength-training regimen to have someone knowledgeable guide our form. There are little changes we can make to how we use our body and/or our weights that make a world of difference. Bad form may not hinder us greatly at first, but once we add power and weight to our exercises, we can really injure our body if we are not working out correctly.

The same is true in our spiritual lives. The Bible gives us so many clues on how to interact with our Heavenly Father more effectively. In fact, Jesus lays out the most basic form in The Lord's Prayer. And when Jesus gives His suggestions, we definitely want to listen.

"Our Father in heaven,
Hallowed be Your name.
Your kingdom come.
Your will be done
On earth as it is in heaven.
Give us day by day our daily bread.
And forgive us our sins,
For we also forgive everyone who is indebted to us.
And do not lead us into temptation,
But deliver us from the evil one."
-Luke 11.2-4 (NKJV)

Good form always starts with making **God's Name holy**. We can praise Him. We can thank Him. We can show Him our highest respect and admiration. Without God, we wouldn't even have the breath in our lungs to whisper a prayer.

Next, we need to be **Kingdom minded**. God has an ultimate plan for our lives, and we can gladly stay open to where He wants to guide our steps every day. Nothing done outside of God's plan will have eternal value, so we should always put His agenda first.

Then, we need to keep our eyes **focused on today**. There are times we will reflect on the past and times we will focus on the future, but most of our time should be spent with our eyes on today. Today is the only day that we can do something for the Lord.

Also, we need to remember that **our sins are forgiven**. When we realize that the price of our sins have been paid by the Finished Work of Jesus on the Cross, we can't help but be joyful. We can have a relationship with God even in our imperfect state because Jesus took our sins and gave us His righteousness.

And since our debt has been forgiven and we have gained everlasting life in heaven, we can **freely forgive others**. This world has been corrupted by sin; so pain, suffering and injustice have entered God's perfect creation. But the heartache won't last long. God will reclaim this world and establish His perfect glory.

Finally, we can **resist temptation**. Temptation is much like lifting weights. God will only allow us to lift the weight of temptation that we can handle. And if the temptation does start to break us, He will do what any good coach will do—He will help carry the burden for us. So we don't have to live in fear. We only need to trust in God. God uses the trials of life to make us spiritually stronger in Him.

"Watch and pray so that you will not fall into temptation. The spirit is willing, but the flesh is weak" *(Matthew 26.41 NIV).*

Chapter 9

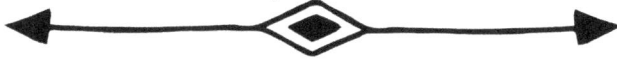

"Better a small serving of vegetables with love than a fattened calf with hatred" (Proverbs 15.17 NIV)

Fitness
Strength Training

It may seem strange, but when we go to the gym to strength train, we are actually going to "break down" muscle. Once we tear the small muscle fibers, they will repair stronger than before as long as we are getting enough protein and the proper amount of nutrition. When we train a particular muscle group, we must let that muscle group rest for several days so it can repair. For this reason, strength trainers will have a weekly routine that works different muscles on different days. Once they break a certain muscle group down, they can focus on a separate muscle group the following day, allowing the first muscle group to rest and restore.

There are **four main avenues of strength training** (also called resistance training). We can use 1) **calisthenics** (our body weight), 2) **strength machines**, 3) **cable machines and bands** and 4) **free weights**. Since we already discussed calisthenics in the HIIT section of the book, we will focus on the last three weight training methods: strength machines, cable machines and bands and free weights. All three methods are great at building muscle and can be integrated into a well-designed work out plan.

Strength machines are readily available at gyms. They are usually easy to use and take less time because the adjustment of weight resistance is fairly simple. They isolate the intended muscle, so we can be sure to add enough weight to work it effectively. Most health clubs will have personal trainers on staff available to teach us how to work these machines. Whenever we join a gym, we need to have a staff member go over each strength machine with us, so we can gain a functional understanding of how they all work. The main disadvantage of strength machines is that they restrain our range of motion. This restraint on our movement prevents us from working the smaller stabilizer muscles that could be involved in the exercise, and the limited movement does not cater to the unique design of each individual.

Cable machines are also at most gyms. They offer resistance training using cables attached to weights. The cables allow us to have a larger range of motion, while still keeping the tension strong. We can do a wide variety of exercises on cable machines and work our muscles in assorted ways. Cable machines are also less time consuming than free weights because we don't have to constantly change out plates, barbells and dumbbells. Cables can be less intimidating than free weights, but they can also seem complicated to a novice. For this reason, it is important to have a personal trainer go over the different exercises on the cable machines. There is a bigger margin of error and more room for injury with cables, so we must take care to keep correct form when using them.

Bands are similar to cable machines, but they use our own body weight and can be done without the bulky machinery. They are very inexpensive and can be done at home. One disadvantage is that bands don't have a heavy resistance load (usually from 8 to 30 pounds). They are good for people who are new to strength training or for people who simply want a good workout at home, the office and/or on vacation.

Free weights are by far the most popular of the strength training methods, but they can be the most intimidating. They allow for free range of movement, they activate the stabilizer muscles and they can work several muscles at once. But walking into a weight room can make us feel apprehensive if we don't know what we are doing. There are a lot of plates, bars, dumbbells, benches, etc., and it all can seem confusing without help. Although most people in a weight room are more than willing to offer assistance and advice, it is important that we have a trainer or coach go over the basics with us first. Good form when working out is imperative, especially when we are loading on the weight. One incorrectly done deadlift can throw out our back for weeks or even months. Also, when increasing muscle mass, we will be working our muscles to fatigue, which is why a workout partner is encouraged. A person "spotting us" will take the weights if our muscles give out, safeguarding us from injury.

Isolated exercises engage one main muscle group in each move, like bicep curls and triceps kickbacks. **Compound exercises** engage more than one major muscle group in each move. The **six major** compound exercises that we definitely want to incorporate into our weight training routine are **bench press, bent over row, squat, dead lift, shoulder press and pull-up or chin-up**. **Pull-ups** and **chip-ups** don't necessarily use free weights (unless they are weighted), but they are a great compound exercise.

1. Bench press works the chest, shoulders and triceps.

2. Bent over row works the back and biceps.

3. Squat works the quadriceps and much of the upper and lower body.

4. Deadlift works the back, hamstrings, gluteus and much of the upper and lower body.

5. Shoulder press works the shoulders and triceps.

6. Pull-up/chin-up works the back and biceps.

We can integrate these six compound moves into our routines along with specifically selected isolated exercises in order to get a full body workout every week. Depending on how many days we want to strength train, we will want to hit all the major muscles groups, including **back, shoulders, chest,**

hamstrings, quadriceps, biceps, triceps and calves. When we work a certain muscle group, we want to make sure we rest it for several days before engaging it fully again. Below are suggested exercises for a one, two and three day strength training routine. We can add isolated exercises to the routines listed by compound exercises. Also, we can integrate **abdominal exercises** throughout our routine or just before our cool down and stretch. The compound exercises do a great job of engaging the abdominals as we brace our core to achieve the exercise.

One Day

Day 1	Full Body Work Out

Two Day

Day 1	Upper Body
Day 2	Lower Body

Two Day
(by compound exercise)

Day 1	Bench Press, Squat, Shoulder Press
Day 2	Dead Lift, Bent Over Row, Pull-up

Three Day

Day 1	Back and hamstrings
Day 2	Quadriceps, calves, chest
Day 3	Shoulders, triceps, biceps

Three Day
(by compound exercise)

Day 1	Bench Press and Squat
Day 2	Dead Lift and Bent Over Row
Day 3	Shoulder Press and Pull-up

Food
Carbohydrates

Carbohydrates are our body's main source of energy. All carbs will be broken down into simple sugars, which is transformed into energy. Carbs are especially important at breakfast time, giving us energy for the day, and directly after our workout, restoring depleted energy. The most popular carbs—corn, rice and wheat—have undergone an unhealthy transformation in our culture. We are taking out most of their nutrients and are pumping them with processed sugar and unhealthy fats. There is really no need to do this since carbs alone are naturally energizing and delicious. When we are choosing carbs to eat, we want to look for the ones that are less processed or even unrefined. Remember, it is not about what we can't have; it's about all the amazing foods we can have.

Refined Carbs vs. Unrefined Carbs

Refined carbs have been manipulated by manufacturers, replacing valuable nutrients with addictive and shelf-preserving additives. When we eat these refined carbs, our body will be filled with empty calories, giving us too much instant energy while starving us nutritionally. We will continue eating the carbs until the bag, box or package is empty, never feeling satiated or satisfied. Unrefined carbs appear much in their natural state and they are filled with nutrients, including much needed fiber.

Unrefined Carbs	Refined Carbs
Whole grains	White sugar
Beans & legumes	Foods with corn syrup
Fresh Fruits	Sodas
Raw vegetables	Sweetened fruit drinks
Oatmeal	White flour
Sweet potatoes	Candy and desserts
Brown & wild rice	White rice

Glycemic Index

All simple carbs are composed of one or two sugar molecules, which cause them to be processed quickly by the body. Carbs that are high on the **Glycemic Index (GI) Scale** are instantly absorbed into the blood stream, elevating our blood sugar. Carbs that are lower on GI Scale are processed slowly and take more time to be absorbed into the blood sugar. Elevated blood sugar releases the insulin hormone, which shuttles the blood sugar to the cells for energy. When we eat too many refined carbs and sugars—candy bars, donuts, sweet rolls, etc.—our blood sugar will spike, giving us a lot of instant energy. However, the insulin released to deal with the sugar overload may cause the blood sugar to drop quickly, leaving us tired and lethargic. Keeping our blood sugar balanced is why we look for carbs that are low to moderate on the GI scale.

Like stated, insulin takes the blood sugar to the cells to be used as energy. However, if we are not exerting the same amount of energy we are consuming, we will have an energy imbalance. If this continues, our insulin will shut down the **body's need to burn fat** and turn on the **body's need to store fat**. We will begin to stockpile fat on our body, especially around our midsection. The best way to lose belly fat is to get our carbs under control. We can kick-start our weight loss with the macro percentage for losing weight (40% protein, 40% fats, 20% carbs), eating mainly fibrous, healthy carbs. Once our insulin is no longer inundated with unused sugars, it will stop storing belly fat. If we work towards having a calorie deficit each day (watching our calorie intake and committing to an exercise routine) we will begin to burn the belly fat.

Simple Carb List

Sugars
Agave Nectar
Honey
Corn Syrup
Molasses
Maple Syrup
Jams
Fruit juices
Gourmet lattes
Candy
Desserts

Healthy Simple Carbs

Whole fruits have a ton of fiber, which causes the body to feel full and aids in digestion. Fruits digest much slower than the other simple carbs, and they are packed full of nutrients. The sugar found in fruit (fructose) comes in smaller doses compared to sugars found in unhealthy simple carbs, like sodas and candy, so they are not as high on the GI chart. Fruit juices have been processed and many times sugar is added in large amounts. The best way to eat fruits is whole and raw. When we feel like we need a sugar fix, we can grab a banana, a handful of grapes or an apple. We can also sweeten foods using fruits and/or juice squeezed directly from the fruits.

Healthy Simple Carbs List

Apples
Bananas
Berries
Nectarines
Plums
Peaches
Pears
Oranges
Melons
Pineapple
Cherries

Complex Carbs (starches)

All complex carbs are composed of sugar molecules that are strung together. Many complex carbs offer much needed fiber and are moderate on the GI Scale. They digest more slowly, so they don't cause an insulin spike. More importantly, they are rich with nutrients and fiber. Starchy and fibrous veggies are both complex carbs. We often forget that vegetables are carbs, but they are the best carbs for us. They are bursting with vitamins and minerals that we can't get from anything else. Plus, they are brimming with fiber. They are low in calories and high in nutrients. We can fill our bellies to the max with veggies, yet still consume fewer calories than what's in a single candy bar. The largest portion on our plate at every meal should always be veggies. A great way to add them to our breakfast is to mix our eggs with onions, peppers, broccoli, tomatoes, spinach, cilantro, etc. Every vegetable is like eating a power-punch of nutrients.

Starchy carbs: potatoes, yams, sweet potatoes, oatmeal, beans, brown rice, peas, pumpkin, barley, quinoa, whole wheat, whole grain

Fibrous carbs: broccoli, spinach, artichokes, green beans, bell peppers, lettuce, tomatoes, Brussels sprouts, onions, mushrooms, carrots, etc.

Fabulous Fiber

Fiber maintains healthy blood sugar levels, aids in digestion and controls appetite. High fiber diets protect the body from heart diseases and certain types of cancer. The recommended daily intake of fiber is between 20 to 45 grams, so we need to add a lot of fibrous foods to our macro carb percentage. Processed carbs won't have the valuable fiber that our body needs, but if we eat an array of veggies along with our unrefined carbs, we will definitely meet our recommended intake of fiber. People who are eating a low percentage of these carbs can get their fill of veggies without exceeding their macro percentage.

High Fiber Foods

Fruits	Serving	Grams of Fiber
Raspberries	1 cup	8.0
Pear	Medium size	5.5
Apple	Medium size	4.4
Banana	Medium size	3.1
Orange	Medium size	3.1
Strawberries	1 cup	3.0
Raisins	60 raisins	1.0

Grains, Cereal & Pasta	Serving	Grams of Fiber
Whole-wheat pasta	1 cup	6.3
Bran flakes	¾ cup	5.3
Oat bran muffin	Medium size	5.2
Oatmeal	1 cup	4.0
Air-popped popcorn	3 cups	3.5
Brown rice	1 cup	3.5
Whole wheat or whole grain bread	1 slice	1.9

Vegetables	Serving	Grams of Fiber
Artichokes	Medium size	10.3
Green peas	1 cup	8.8
Broccoli	1 cup	5.1
Brussels Sprouts	1 cup	4.1
Corn	1 cup	4.0
Potato	Small size	3.0
Carrots	Medium size	1.7

Nuts, Legumes & Seeds	Serving	Grams of Fiber
Lentils	1 cup	15.6
Black beans	1 cup	15.0
Baked beans	1 cup	10.4
Sunflower seeds	¼ cup	3.9
Almonds	23 nuts	3.5
Pistachios	49 nuts	2.9
Pecans	10 whole	2.7

Faith
Muscle Contraction

"'Love the Lord your God with all your heart and with all your soul and with all your mind and with all your strength.' The second is this: 'Love your neighbor as yourself.' There is no commandment greater than these" (Mark 12.30-31 NIV).

The muscles in our body have three types of contraction: **Concentric Contraction, Eccentric Contraction** and **Isometric Contraction.** These combined contractions allow our effectively designed body to perform and accomplish amazing tasks.

During **Concentric Contraction**, the muscle shortens and comes together to overcome a certain resistance. An example of this type of contraction is how the bicep contracts to lift the weight of a dumbbell curl.

During **Eccentric Contraction**, the muscle lengthens as it contracts to control and/or stop a movement. An example of this type of contraction is how the bicep lengthens as it safely brings the weight of the dumbbell back down from a curl.

During **Isometric Contraction**, the muscle resists movement, stabilizing itself under intense pressure, while the body remains firm. An example of this type of contraction is how the core of the body maintains the tense position of a plank without moving.

All three of these muscle contractions are important to exercise, especially strength training. Compound exercises, like deadlifts, use all three muscle contractions. Concentric and eccentric contractions are used when the weight of the bar is being lifted and brought back down, and the core muscles are stabilizing the body during the dead lift in an isometric contraction, keeping the body in perfect form. Without all three contractions, the compound exercise could not be done. The awesome benefit of compound exercises is that a maximum number of muscle groups are being engaged simultaneously during all three muscle contractions, which builds muscle throughout the body much faster.

Our faith muscles also have three contractions. God gives us each promises in this life, and He expects us to build our spiritual muscles in order to move them into reality. God has given us free will, and though we need His supernatural help to achieve our promises, He still expects us to move our spiritual muscles by faith. God is our Master Trainer, and He wants us to be strong in Christ. He won't take the weight from us when He knows that we are fully capable of maintaining it.

"For no matter how many promises God has made, **they are "Yes" in Christ.** *And so through him the "Amen" is spoken by us to the glory of God"* (2 Corinthians 1.20 NIV).

A **Spiritual Concentric Contraction** occurs when God allows resistance on our path to claiming our promises. If our promises were easy to achieve, we wouldn't grow to reach them, and we would probably take them for granted. God expects us to squeeze tight, giving every ounce of energy we have to bring those dreams to fruition. It may take years of squeezing and trying, but the promises are "yes" in Christ. We need only to continue building our muscle.

*"Let us not become weary in doing good, for at the proper time we will reap a harvest **if we do not give up**" (Galatians 6.9 NIV).*

A **Spiritual Eccentric Contraction** occurs when we resist the temptations of a world controlled by Satan. Satan hates humans with an intense, supernatural hatred, and all he wants do is "steal, kill and destroy" everything to do with humanity (John 10.10). When we resist the devil, we are wielding great amount of strength. However, the best way to not allow that tension to break us is to keep our eyes on our Master Trainer. He won't give us any resistance that He knows that we won't be able to withstand.

*"No temptation has overtaken you except what is common to mankind. And God is faithful; **he will not let you be tempted beyond what you can bear.** But when you are tempted, he will also provide a way out so that you can endure it" (1 Corinthians 10.13 NIV).*

A **Spiritual Isometric Contraction** occurs when we stand firm. Sometimes God gets quiet in our lives, and we feel like we have no immediate direction. When this occurs, we need to do a spiritual plank, staying rigid in our faith. Often times we are so productive-oriented that we don't like being still, but what we need to realize is that God is working our spiritual muscles in an Isometric Contraction. He wants us to hold the position and wait on His next command, not moving to the left or to the right (Proverbs 4.27). He wants to see if we will stand firmly on His promises and wait patiently, activating our faith muscles according to His time and will.

*"Be on your guard; **stand firm in the faith**; be courageous; be strong" (1 Corinthians 16.13 NIV).*

God wants us to grow and strengthen in Him, so He will allow seasons of "compound exercises" in our life that activate all three contractions: Concentric, Eccentric and Isometric. These times may be difficult to bear, but God is our Master Training, and He is shaping us into the image of His Perfect Son, Jesus. We are becoming the people we will be for eternity, and God wants to exercise our faith, so we can grow strong in Him. But don't worry, like any good trainer, God will give us a time of rest, so our sore, torn muscles can repair and become even stronger than before.

*"But those who trust in the Lord will find **new strength**.*
They will soar high on wings like eagles.
They will run and not grow weary.
They will walk and not faint."
    – Isaiah 40.31 (NLT).

Chapter 10

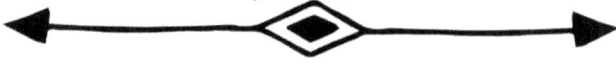

"No discipline is enjoyable while it is happening—it's painful. But afterward there will be a peaceful harvest of right living for those who are trained in this way" (Hebrews 12.11 NLT).

Fitness
Slow-twitch/Fast-twitch Muscle Fibers

Slow-twitch muscle fibers contract slowly and are mainly used in aerobic exercises that are low intensity. They create repetitive and steady contractions that we use when we are jogging, cycling, swimming, etc. Fast-twitch muscle fibers contract quickly and are mainly used in anaerobic exercises that are high intensity. They are used in short, intense bursts when we are sprinting, playing sports or lifting weights. The more we do of aerobic exercises, the stronger our slow-twitch fibers become. The more we do anaerobic exercises, the stronger our fast-twitch muscle fibers become.

For this reason, when people are training for an aerobic competition, like the Boston Marathon, Ironman or Grand Tour (cycling), they want to focus on strengthening their slow-twitch muscles fibers. Therefore, they probably won't be seen in the weight room, squatting 500 pounds. The same goes for people training for an anaerobic competition, like a sport or bodybuilding competition, they want to focus on strengthening their fast-twitch muscle fibers. Therefore, we usually won't see them running their 20th mile on the track.

Most of us, however, can work both muscle fibers for a more balanced fitness experience. We usually won't reach the extremes of a 500-pound squat or a 26-mile run unless we have set it as a goal. Setting goals is an awesome way to stay motivated; otherwise, our motivation will be to maintain a personal level of health and fitness. However, each body type may be predisposed to certain activities because of its design and build. We may find certain activities easier to do than others and that we excel more quickly doing them. Our body type can actually encourage us into different areas of exercise because they are more enjoyable for us. We will discuss the body types and their related exercises in the next chapter.

Food
Fats

The two main sources of fats are **saturated fats** and **unsaturated fats**. Fats are condensed energy that help hormone production in the body, help with making our cell membranes, help with developing our nervous system and help carry fat-soluble vitamins through the body. Saturated fats are no worse or better than unsaturated fats; however, we are consuming more saturated fats because we are eating fewer plants and fish and more animal products, which creates an unhealthy imbalance. Saturated fats include butter, animal fats and coconut oil. Unsaturated fats can be divided into two categories: **polyunsaturated fats** and **monounsaturated fats**. Polyunsaturated fats include **Omega 3** (from flaxseed, fish and walnut oil) and **Omega 6** (from corn oil, sunflower oil and peanut oil). Monounsaturated fats come from olive oil and avocado oil.

Another unhealthy imbalance we face today is seen in our Omega 3 and Omega 6 intake. We are consuming too much Omega 6, mainly because our culture widely uses **corn and peanuts** as vegetable oils for cooking. And we don't consume enough Omega 3 because we don't eat enough fish, flaxseeds and walnuts as much. We can correct this problem by simply eating more fish, by adding flaxseed to foods, by cooking with alternative oils, like walnut oil, and by using less vegetable oils with corn and peanuts.

There is one fat that we should avoid—**trans fats**. Trans fats are unsaturated fats that have been processed by adding hydrogen to vegetable oil, causing the oil to become solid at room temperature, increasing the shelf life. Trans fats are in almost anything processed: **baked goods**, like cakes, frostings, pie crusts, crackers, cookies, canned dough and pizza crusts; **snacks**, like potato chips, corn chips and microwaveable popcorn; and **fried foods**, like French fries, donuts and breaded and fried meats and vegetables. When we read that list, we realize just how many of those food items our generation is eating, and the trend is being passed on to the next generation. Most kid menu items at restaurants are filled with processed carbs, processed meats, trans fats and sugar-laden drinks, so we have to take care to seek out alternatives. For example, instead of ordering a corn dog and fries, we can order grilled chicken and apple slices.

Fats can be overwhelming and confusing, but safe to say, if we are eating healthy foods, staying under our calorie limit and consuming our macro percentages, we should have a balanced diet. We don't need to know everything all at once. We can slowly gain information about healthy eating and apply it naturally. Ransacking our kitchen, throwing away everything out of fear and guilt, doesn't fix the problem. It is best to simply make a few changes at a time and apply them. Once those changes become incorporated into our new healthy lifestyle, we can make a few more changes and apply them. Before we know it, all the foods we wanted to throw out will soon be replaced by healthier varieties—and we won't have an empty pantry and refrigerator.

Faith
The Power of Tearing Down

"Come, let us return to the LORD. He has torn us to pieces but he will heal us; he has injured us but he will bind up our wounds" (Hosea 6.1 NIV).

When we go to the gym to lift weights, we are actually going to break down muscle by tearing the muscle fibers. We know that unless we are lifting heavy, we won't create muscle hypertrophy (increasing muscle mass). Once we tear down our muscles by lifting loads that are almost too heavy for us, we have to allow those muscles to rest. As they rest, our muscles repair themselves even bigger and stronger than before.

"Come to me, all you who are weary and burdened, and I will give you rest" (Matthew 11.28 NIV).

When we go back to the gym to work the same muscle group, the weight that was once almost too heavy now becomes bearable. And after it becomes bearable, it will become easy. When the weight becomes too easy, we will have to add more pounds to make the weight almost too heavy again. It is amazing how quickly the body can adapt to the pressure placed on it. God's ingenious design of our body allows us to gain as much muscle mass that we are willing to tear down.

"So do not fear, for I am with you; do not be dismayed, for I am your God. I will strengthen you and help you; I will uphold you with my righteous right hand" (Isaiah

41.10 NIV).

When people hear that God will tear them down, many of them don't understand. They wonder if God is good, why would He willingly break us? If God loves us, why would He want us to suffer? These are questions that are limited to a temporal understanding; they don't take into consideration an eternal point-of-view. God has us on the earth for a reason, and it's definitely not to coast through blissfully until we see Jesus face-to-face in Heaven.

"So we fix our eyes not on what is seen, but on what is unseen, since what is seen is temporary, but what is unseen is eternal" (2 Corinthians 4.18 NIV).

God is more concerned about the people we will be for eternity, and He is using this world to tear us down, so He can build us back up stronger in Him. He wants us to do amazing feats for His glory, but if we are too weak, we will buckle under the pressure. Each of God's blessings come with a burden. And God will withhold that blessing until we are strong enough to stand under the weight that comes with it.

"Dear brothers and sisters, when troubles of any kind come your way, consider it an opportunity for great joy. For you know that when your faith is tested, your endurance has a chance to grow. So let it grow, for when your endurance is fully developed, you will be perfect and complete, needing nothing" (James 1.2-4 NLT).

God desires that we become so "fully developed" that we will be "perfect and complete, needing nothing." Our spiritual strength is built when God breaks down our preconceived notions of our own strength, forcing us to rely solely on His. When God is our complete strength, we will indeed be "needing nothing." Since God is the Creator and Owner of everything, our total reliance on Him will create a portal, giving us everything we need when we need it.

"And my God will meet all your needs according to the riches of his glory in Christ Jesus" (Philippians 4.19 NIV).

So when we leave the gym knowing that we have torn our muscle fibers, we should be very pleased. We've accomplished what we set out to do, and we are on our way to gaining the strength and muscle mass we are wanting. If we were to run away from the pain and suffering, we would never become physically stronger. We know that when we enter into the gym, we will experience brokenness, but the breaking is what causes healing, which leads to gained strength.

"For he wounds, but he also binds up; he injures, but his hands also heal" (Job 5.18 NIV).

The same is true for life. Life is like a gym–we engage knowing that we will experience pain and suffering, but that does not mean we should continually run away from hardships. Pain is part of the process of growth, and God is near us when we are broken. He is repairing us into the image of Christ, so we can become our best selves and accomplish the purposes that God has planned for us.

"The Lord is close to the brokenhearted; he rescues those whose spirits are crushed" (Psalm 34.18 NLT).

Chapter 11

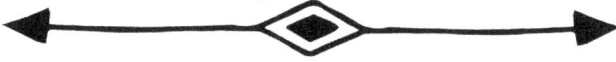

"Search for the Lord and for his strength; continually seek him" (1 Chronicles 16.11 NLT).

Fitness
Exercise for Body types

Knowing our body type will help us understand the characteristics of our body better, making it easier for us to form realistic fitness goals. These three body types are not the end-all and say-all in our body design, but they are here to help guide us into developing a fitness program to suit our needs. Below is a possible list of exercises for the three body types and some explanations. However, we must all form our own opinions based on our desires and experiences. We can listen to suggestions, but we must apply only the information that feels right for us.

Ectomorphs have high metabolisms and have long and lean muscles, so gaining muscle bulk is difficult for them. If ectomorphs want to achieve more muscle mass, they will have to focus most of their attention in the weight room and consume more calories to compensate for their high metabolisms. Otherwise, they do well with light resistance training and a few days of aerobic exercise—running, swimming, cycling, etc.—every week. They can also excel in yoga and Pilates classes because of their long muscles and their high metabolism, which allows them to do low-intensity workouts and still stay slender.

Mesomorphs have an athletic build and can gain and lose weight easily. They build muscle quickly and effectively, so they can do a few days of strength training and/or HIIT and maintain a fit figure. They do well in aerobics classes and can even do long stretches of cardio on machines—treadmill, stair stepper, rowing machine, etc. If they are aerobically in shape, they may excel in playing sports, so joining an amateur sport's league may help them reach their fitness goals.

Endomorphs have lower metabolisms, so they may have to focus on extended periods of aerobic exercise to lose any excess weight. Water aerobics is great for endomorphs who are just starting up their exercise routine. Cardio sessions of about 40 minutes 3-5 times a week will help boost their metabolism, and once they became aerobically strong, they can begin doing HIIT with their cardio sessions. Endomorphs have naturally solid muscles, so strength training could definitely be a goal for them, especially since their protein macro is high.

What are some of your favorite exercise routines?

Food
Combining Macros

We want to eat all three macros—carbohydrates, proteins and fats—at every meal, according to the percentage of our body type. The morning time and right after we exercise are the best times for the complex carbohydrates, like oat, rice and whole grain. Later on in the day, we can rely more on fibrous vegetables (broccoli, spinach and salads) to meet our carb macro. We should also avoid eating heavy, fatty foods (salmon, steak, dairy) right after we exercise because they will slow down digestion, delaying much needed energy from getting into our muscles. We need quick energy to repair and sustain our muscles after we work out, so a rice cake or sweet potato would be perfect.

Our perception of portion size may also be a little off because most restaurants serve double to triple the portion size. We may even have adapted this portion overload in our own homes. In the beginning, we may have to buy and use a food scale and measuring cups to ensure that the amount we eat matches what we are inputting into our calorie counter. Once we get accustomed to eyeballing the correct quantity, we won't have to weigh or measure our foods very often. Below is a list of foods and their recommended portion size. We usually eat a little over the portion size, but as long as we are adding the correct ounces to our calorie counter, we will be able to keep track of the calories we are consuming.

Grains: 1 slice of whole grain bread, 1 cup dry cereal, ½ cup cooked oatmeal, pasta or rice. A pancake should like a CD and a bagel should look like a 6 oz. can of tuna.

Meats: 3 oz. of lean meat or poultry is like the palm of our hand. 3 oz. of grilled fish is like a checkbook.

Fruits: 1 medium whole fruit or ½ cup of sliced fruit.

Vegetables: 1 cup of leafy vegetables or ½ cup of sliced vegetables.

Nuts, seeds and legumes: 1/3 cups nuts, 2 tablespoons peanut butter or seeds, ½ cup dried beans or peas.

Dairy: 1 cup of milk, 1 cup of yogurt, 1 & ½ cup of cottage cheese.

Fats and oils: 1 tablespoon.

Breakfast

Breakfast is a very important meal and should not be skipped. Eating within the first hour we awake will boost our metabolism and give us the energy we need to start our day. Also, eating breakfast will prevent our blood sugar from getting too low, which may make us overeat when we finally consume our first meal. Processed meats are prolific during breakfast (sausage, bacon, ham). We can look for healthier options that are lower in sodium and are made without nitrates. Even better, we can dice up the steak, turkey or lean pork from the night before and mixed that with our eggs, making a very delicious and nutritious omelet.

Breakfast Example 1

An example of a healthy breakfast would be a buckwheat pancake with blueberries, one egg and one portion of egg whites mixed with peppers, onions and tomatoes cooked with a small drizzle of walnut oil.

Carbohydrates	Proteins	Fats
Buckwheat pancake Blueberries Peppers Onions Tomatoes	1 egg, 1 portion egg whites	Walnut oil

Breakfast Example 1 = 400 calories, 13g of fat, 41g of carbs, 17.5 grams of protein and 8 grams of fiber.

Breakfast Example 2

Another example of a healthy breakfast would be 1/2 cup of steel cut oats with a sprinkle of flaxseed and 1/3 cup of diced apples and 3/4 cup of low fat Greek yogurt mixed with 1/4 cup of walnuts.

Carbohydrates	Proteins	Fats
1/2 cup of steel cut oats 1/3 cup diced apples	3/4 cup of Greek yogurt (low fat)	1/4 cup of Walnuts Sprinkle of flaxseed

Breakfast Example 2 = 400 calories, 16g of fat, 34g of carbs, 30g of protein and 5 grams of fiber.

Lunch

Lunch is when we need to pay close attention to our eating. Many of us go out to eat for lunch and consume the rest of the day's calories in one meal. We need to look for lighter and smaller portion choices or we can bring a lunch from home. If we want to use half our lunch hour for aerobic exercise, a small, healthy lunch that can be eaten quickly would be a wise choice. Endomorphs should always be looking for alternatives to higher carb items. A good replacement for rice is broccoli. Broccoli is lower on the **Glycemic Index Scale** and has much fewer calories. Plus, broccoli is crunchy and mixes well with most foods.

Also, we don't have to get rid of our favorite salad dressings to avoid extra calories. We simply need to eat less of it. We can ask for the salad dressing on the side, and dip each forkful of salad into our dressing before each bite. We'll be surprised to see half our salad dressing left in the cup when we are done. And sandwiches are the sneakiest calorie collectors on the lunch menu, but we don't have to avoid them. We simply need to ask for no bun. If we can get large strips of romaine lettuce on the side, we can make a lettuce wrap with any sandwich on the menu. An Italian roast beef sandwich is amazing wrapped in sweet, crispy romaine lettuce.

Lunch Example 1

An example lunch would be 4 oz. chicken breast, 1/4 cup sliced avocado, 1/2 cup of brown rice (or 1 cup of broccoli) and a small salad (no croutons) with the salad dressing on the side.

Carbohydrate	Proteins	Fats
1/2 cup of Brown rice (or 1 cup of broccoli) Side salad	4 oz. Chicken breast.	1/4 avocado Salad dressing

Lunch Example 1 (with rice) = 430 calories, 14.5g fat, 29.5g of carbs, 39g of protein and 2.6g of fiber.

Lunch Example 1 (with broccoli) = 350 calories, 14g fat, 13g of carbs, 39.5g of protein and 3g of fiber.

Lunch Example 2

Another example of a healthy lunch would be a sandwich with whole grain bread (or romaine lettuce for a wrap), 3 oz. turkey breast, one slice of low-fat Swiss cheese, onion and tomato with 2 tablespoons of hummus and 1/2 cup of sliced bell pepper on the side.

Carbohydrate	Protein	Fats
Whole grain bread (or romaine lettuce) Tomato Onion Bell Pepper	3 oz. sliced Turkey 2 Tablespoons Hummus	One slice low fat Swiss cheese

Lunch Example 2 (with whole grain bread) = 480 calories, 13g fat, 60g of carbs, 36.5g of protein and 11g of fiber.

Lunch Example 2 (with romaine lettuce for wrap) = 310 calories, 11g of fat, 25.5g of carbs, 28g of protein and 9g of fiber.

Dinner

Dinner is the time that we want to cut out the complex carbs and load up on fibrous veggies. A good rule of thumb is to make a lean portion of meat with a side or two of fibrous vegetables for dinner. Casseroles, pastas, breads and potatoes are not necessary to have a fantastic meal. We can save those items for post-work out lunch or for our "cheat meals," which will be discussed chapter 14. Instead, we can add a little more fats to our dinner, getting creative with light sauces for our meats and vegetables. We also need to watch our portion size at dinner. One portion of meat is about the size of our palm. This is why we should fill our plates to overflowing with veggies—they will fill our bellies with nutritional, low calorie goodness.

To get ahead on the time it takes to cook dinner, It's a good idea to cook or barbeque all our meat for the entire week. This way we can be sure to cook lean meats and not have to worry about rushing. Many of us eat low quality, high calorie foods when we are busy, but if we cook our meat for the week ahead of time, we won't have to compromise. We can use this lean meat for our breakfast instead of the highly processed breakfast meat that's usually available. We can also add this meat to a side of brown rice for lunch. At one time, we can cook a ham, pork chops, steaks, chicken, salmon, tilapia, etc. and have our protein read for when we need it.

Dinner Example 1

5 oz. filet mignon, 1/2 cup of creamed spinach and 1 cup of garlic and onion roasted Brussels sprouts in olive oil.

Carbohydrate	Protein	Fats
Spinach Brussels sprouts Onion Garlic	5 oz. filet mignon	Creamed cheese Olive oil

Dinner Example 1 = 425 calories, 23g of fat, 6g of carbs, 34g of protein and 5g of fiber.

Dinner Example 2

Another example of a healthy dinner is 4 oz. lean beef and 1/4 cup of low fat feta cheese stuffed bell pepper,

Caesar salad with tomatoes and 1 tablespoon of parmesan cheese.

Carbohydrate	Protein	Fats
1 bell pepper 1 cup of romaine lettuce 6 cherry tomatoes	4 oz. Lean beef	1 tablespoon of parmesan cheese ¼ cup feta cheese Caesar dressing

Dinner Example 2 = 420 calories, 20g of fat, 18g of carbs, 40g of protein and 3g of fiber.

These examples of healthy meals are only a few of the thousands of delicious meal ideas found online and in bookstores. Today, like no other time in history, we have a wealth of healthy resources at our disposal. All we have to do is take time to learn them, use them and make them healthy staples at our mealtime. Also, we will notice that exchanging our starchy carbs (bread and rice) for fibrous veggie alternatives (broccoli and romaine lettuce) makes a vast difference in our calorie intake. If we know we are going to eat a lot of carbs at lunch, we can adjust our breakfast macros to compensate. **That's what makes eating according to our macros so amazing—we can adjust them to fit our needs.**

Grazing: Eating Six Times a Day

Three meals a day might be easier to fit into our schedule, but our body benefits from eating six smaller meals every 2-4 hours. When the body realizes that it is being fed consistently, it will be better able to let go of fat stores being saved for dire situations (starving). Also, regular feedings keep our metabolism going at a steady rate and keep our blood sugar from dropping too low (causing us to feel hungry and binge eat). Another benefit of eating every few hours is that there is no pressure to eat like it's the "last meal." The mind knows that the body will be fed again in a few hours, so there is no need to overeat.

With our three meals a day, we can add 3 small snacks: **between breakfast and lunch**, **between lunch and dinner** and **right before bed**. This will give us 6 feedings a day. We may fear that we will overeat with all these meals, but the truth is that if we are eating low calorie and high nutritional foods, **we will actually be eating much more, yet consuming fewer calories.** The snack before bedtime is very important. Many of us overeat at dinnertime, but if we realize we are going to get a small snack before bed, we won't feel the urge to stuff our bellies. But before we start eating our snacks, we need to take off 100-150 calories from each of our meals. If we are eating healthy foods, this won't be hard. And if we are working out, it will be even easier.

Good snacks include, ½ cup of low-fat cottage cheese with pineapple, ¼ cup of almonds, apple with 1 tablespoon of peanut butter, cup of almond milk with whey protein, Greek yogurt with granola, carrot sticks and low-fat ranch and grapes with a small cheese wedge.

Faith
The Power of Muscle Balance

"We can rejoice, too, when we run into problems and trials, for we know that they help us develop endurance. And endurance develops strength of character, and character strengthens our confident hope of salvation" (Romans 5.3-4 NLT).

Muscle imbalance means that some of our muscle groups are stronger than others. This causes an imbalance in our body that can hinder training. **1)** Stronger muscles will compensate for weaker ones, which causes the stronger ones to strain and the weaker ones to atrophy (become weaker). **2)** The body's form will be sabotaged during workouts, since the stronger muscles will adjust to counteract the weaker ones. **3)** The stronger muscles will begin to wear and tear from overuse because of incorrect form and usage. **4)** The amount of weight lifted will be compromised, since all muscles (especially in compound exercises) are not being fully activated.

"But the Holy Spirit produces this kind of fruit in our lives: love, joy, peace, patience, kindness, goodness, faithfulness, gentleness, and self-control. There is no law against these things." (Galatians 5.22-23 NLT).

We also have spiritual muscles. Our spiritual muscles include **love, joy, peace, patience, kindness, goodness, faithfulness, gentleness** and **self-control.** When we go into the gym of life, we will have faith muscle imbalance. God has given us the Fruits of the Spirit because of Jesus' Finished Work on the Cross, but we have to activate and grow them in our lives. God does not want us to be imbalanced. He wants us to have the fullness of all His fruit because Jesus died to give them to us. God is training us to become the people we will be for eternity, and He wants all of our faith muscles to be strong.

If we are weak in one of the spiritual fruits (e.g. patience or self-control), our stronger spiritual fruit (e.g. peace and goodness) may try to compensate. We may be able to handle a short time under small amounts of resistance, but when the weight gets really heavy, we could possibly lose form and buckle under the pressure. It's good to have strengths, but when it comes to the Fruits of the Spirit, God wants us to be strong in all areas. God will place weight (difficulty, trials, tribulation) in our lives to help build those faith muscles. Yes, the weight will be difficult, and the pain will create soreness or even pain; but God is the Loving Trainer, encouraging us to press forward and push harder. God wants us to attain complete spiritual muscle hypertrophy, so we will be fully strong for Him.

So the next time we enter into the gym of life, we don't have to be scared about the weight and the struggle. God is watching over us. None of our pain and suffering goes to waste—they are each shaping us into the spiritually fit powerhouse that God wants us to become. We must not shy away from the Fruits of the Holy Spirit that are the hardest for us to strengthen. We can embrace them, knowing that they are becoming stronger with every trial we face and overcome. God wants us to be heavyweight champions for Him, and He will build up all of our spiritual muscle if we let Him.

"The name of the Lord is a strong tower; the righteous man runs into it and is safe" (Proverbs 18.10 ESV).

Chapter 12

---◆---

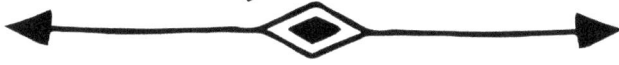

"Enlarge the place of your tent, stretch your tent curtains wide, do not hold back; lengthen your cords, strengthen your stakes" (Isaiah 54.2 NIV).

Fitness
Warm Up, Cool Down and Stretching

Although exercise prevents injury by keeping our bones, muscles, ligaments and tendons strong, it can also cause injury if we are not careful. There is a risk of doing any activity, but we can be proactive about staying safe if we follow a few simple suggestions. Many times our warm up, cool down and stretches go to the wayside because we don't value them as much as the actual workout. But if we take time to do them, we will find that our exercise routine will benefit greatly.

Warm Up

A five-minute warm up before we start a rigorous exercise routine is very important, especially if our goal is to hit a higher target heart rate or even our max heart rate. The warm up increases body temperature, warming up our muscles and connective tissues. It increases the blood flow to the heart and muscles, bringing the necessary oxygen and nutrients. It prepares the cardiopulmonary system for the forthcoming workload. And it readies the mind, equipping us with the will to dominate our workout.

Cool Down

A five-minute cool down after we've just completed a demanding exercise routine, soothes the body gently back to a relaxing state. If we have just finished a High Intensity Interval Training (HIIT) workout, our heart rate can be at its limit, so we need to allow it time to slowly come back down. Plus, we may have lactic acid built up in our muscles and bloodstream, and our body needs time to process that waste material. A cool down is like allowing a racecar that has just been going 200 mph to gradually roll to a stop, instead of simply slamming on the breaks. Slamming on the breaks after hitting max speeds can be devastating to a car, and we are no less different. The systems in our body have been working overtime to keep up with our intense workout, so they need time to run normally again. And we too probably have to regain our composure after pushing our body to the limit before we jump to the next portion of our day.

Stretching

Stretching is one of the most undervalued aspects of our exercise routine. Our muscles are getting stronger and stronger, yet they are become tighter and tighter because we aren't flexible. Stretching—along with proper form—is one of the main ways to prevent injury. Stretching keeps our muscles and connective tissues durable and pliable, which is important when we are lifting heavy loads or doing powerful bursts of movements. Everything in our body is connected, so if one area of our body is tight, it will affect the other areas. For example, if we are suffering from lower back pain, it may be because our hamstrings are too tight. Also, without adequate flexibility, our posture will be compromised and our form during many strength-training exercises, like the squat, will suffer. If our hip flexors are tight, we won't be able to do a full squat. We can incorporate stretching into our warm up and/or cool down to prevent injury and to help us feel and do our best.

Food
Importance of Water

Water is extremely important to our body. In fact, without water we would die in just a few days. Having barely enough water every day ensures that our body can survive, but when we have an abundance of water, our body will thrive. Although our body is composed of around 60% water, the water is not evenly distributed. Some of the most important parts of our body are made up of mostly water: our brain is 85%, our blood is 80% and our muscles are 70% water. Drinking our recommended amount of water each day will maintain the health of these vital body components.

We need daily intakes of water to keep the systems and functions of our body working properly, including digestion, circulation, transportation of nutrients and maintenance of body temperature—just to name a few. When our body is functioning properly, we are functioning properly. Water also helps our organs work smoothly, including our kidneys and our gastrointestinal (GI) tract. Plus, water keeps our skin, hair and nails looking and feeling great, making it the cheapest beauty product on the market today.

Water also reduces the chance of illness because it helps our body to easily flush out waste material, like toxins, and transport healthy nutrients to our cells. If we are consuming water and eating a bunch of amazingly nutritious fruits and vegetables at every meal, our blood stream will be flowing with vitamins and minerals just waiting to feed our cells. Water keeps us healthy at the cellular level, which will ensure a vigorous immune system, keeping us strong to fight against illness and disease.

Water also can help us lose weight because many times we confuse our thirst signal for a hunger signal, and we eat unnecessary calories trying to quench our thirst. Water actually can suppress our appetite, so before we go into the pantry for a snack, we should gulp down a big glass of water. Plus, when we drink water at every meal instead of sugar-laden sodas, juices or teas, we will save our body from consuming a ton of empty calories that offer no nutritional benefits. According to the Mayo Clinic, men should drink **13 cups** of water a day and woman should drink **9 cups** of water a day. However, if we are committed to a rigorous workout regiment and/or we live in a hot and humid location, we can drink upwards to **16-24 cups** of water a day (1 gallon to 1 & ½ gallon).

Faith
The Power of Living Water

"But those who drink the water I give will never be thirsty again. It becomes a fresh, bubbling spring within them, giving them eternal life" (John 4.14 NLT).

We first drink of Living Water when we receive salvation through Jesus Christ and His Finished Work on the Cross. However, it is up to us to daily drink of the Living Water that is freely given to us. There are many ways to drink in Living Water, but the two largest available wellsprings are found in the Bible and the Holy Spirit.

The Bible says that Jesus was the Word made Flesh. Jesus walked this earth, but He has been writing His message through the lives of His Children since the beginning of time. His words are found in the 66 books of the Bible. The Bible is a collection of stories about different people during various times, but the theme throughout every page and verse reflects Jesus.

"The Word became flesh and made his dwelling among us. We have seen his glory, the glory of the one and only Son, who came from the Father, full of grace and truth" (John 1.14 NIV).

When we consume the Bible, we are literally allowing Jesus, the Living Water, to pour into our spiritual lives. And our spiritual well-being affects every aspect of our life on earth–mind, body, heart and soul. We must intake daily doses of God's Word, so the functions of our life run smoothly and stay strong under pressure. (God allows "pressure" in our lives because He's growing our spiritual muscles.) The Holy Spirit in each of us unlocks the living aspect of the Bible, and we start to transform under its influence.

"For the word of God is alive and powerful. It is sharper than the sharpest two-edged sword, cutting between soul and spirit, between joint and marrow. It exposes our innermost thoughts and desires" (Hebrews 4.12 NLT).

The Holy Spirit is the other fountain of Living Water available to us. Jesus died on the Cross in order to forgive the sins of the world, so we could have God's Spirit inside of us. The Holy Spirit's presence in our life is proof that Jesus' Work on the Cross accomplished the reconciliation of humanity. (We were separated by sin because of our free will choices of disobedience.) Jesus died, taking our sins with Him, but He took back up His life, leaving sin behind. This Truth allows us to have a relationship with the Holy Spirit even in our imperfect state because by grace we receive salvation and by faith we are righteous before a Holy God.

"(When he said 'living water,' he was speaking of the Spirit, who would be given to everyone believing in him. But the Spirit had not yet been given, because Jesus had not yet entered into his glory.)" (John 7.39 NLT).

When we spend time with the Holy Spirit in prayer, we are drinking up large amounts of Living Water. God loves us, and He did not leave us alone. He died to be with us while we were yet sinners (Romans 5.8). Sitting in prayer may be difficult at first, but once we notice the amazing benefits of spending time with God, we will become addicted. God's Spirit will guide us in all truth (John 16.13).

Moreover, we will begin to learn to distinguish God's voice and listen for it throughout our day. We'll become accustomed to His presence, and He will work alongside the Bible to accomplish His amazing will in our life. We'll begin to see a difference in our outlook, and the pressures that once tried to destroy us will now be manageable. We were not created to live without our Heavenly Father. We need His Living Water in our lives every moment of the day. The Living Water is pouring forth–all we need to do is drink deeply.

"Anyone who believes in me may come and drink. For the Scriptures declare, 'Rivers of living water will flow from his heart'" (John 7.38 NLT).

Chapter 13

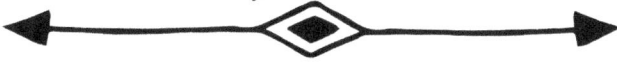

"*Let us then approach God's throne of grace with confidence, so that we may receive mercy and find grace to help us in our time of need*" *(Hebrews 4.16 NIV).*

Fitness
Personal Trainer

When we decide that we want to take our health and fitness to the next level, hiring a personal trainer (Certified Fitness Trainer) for a few months will be well worth the investment. Personal trainers have been trained to work with all types of people, helping them to grow in their fitness knowledge and strength. Personal trainers can help motivate us and equip us to achieve the fitness goals that we have set and to overcome all the obstacles standing in our way. They can give us the confidence and reassurance we need to make that next step in our fitness lifestyle.

There are five main personal training programs available:

1. American Council on Exercise (**ACE**)

2. American College of Sports Medicine (**ACSM**)

3. International Sports Sciences Association (**ISSA**)

4. National Academy of Sports Medicine (**NASM**)

5. National Strength and Conditioning Association (**NSCA**)

Each of the certification programs works diligently to ensure that they are preparing their students to help their clients achieve fitness success. However, there are some key characteristics that we want to look for before choosing a personal trainer.

1) **Education**: Not only do we want our trainers to be certified in a program, we want them to keep up with new and relevant information in the fitness and health field. We want to look for trainers who are always reading books, posts and articles, so they can continue to improve their knowledge and ability.

2) **Experience:** Unless we are allowing new trainers to learn on our time, we definitely want trainers who have experience. We can ask for letters of recommendation, we can look at before and after pictures of previous clients and we can talk with the managing staff of the gym that we attend.

3) **Organized:** Our time is limited, and we want personal trainers who are prepared at every

session. Our trainers should be punctual and ready with our nutritional and fitness plans on time.

4) **Professional:** If personal trainers don't take their job seriously, there is no reason for us to waste our time and money. Trainers should look like they belong in a gym, and they should always treat their clients with respect and care.

5) **Personality:** If we don't get along with certain personal trainers, it doesn't matter how much education or experience they have. We must feel comfortable if we are going to excel under their guidance, so we need to make sure to find people we work well with.

Food
Insulin Resistance

The GI Index is the rate at which consumed carbs raise the blood sugar and signal the release of insulin in the body. It is best to have high GI foods in the morning, so we can have energy for the day. Then we can have high GI foods after our work out, so insulin can bring energy (broken down sugars from carbs) to the muscle for rapid repair. The function of carbs bringing energy to the cells is a very effective design; however, we are sabotaging this design by overeating energy and not exerting enough energy.

When we consume too much energy, we begin storing excess fat (especially belly fat) in our body, but after a while, we may become insulin resistant, which is the precursor to Type II Diabetes. There are projections that in just one decade almost half the population of America will be diabetic or pre-diabetic. We are eating so much processed carbs and sugars that our blood sugar is becoming thick with energy with absolutely nowhere to go. Unless we are running a marathon every day, there is no need for so much energy.

When we become insulin resistant, our cells no longer respond to the overload of insulin that has been released over and over again through the years of overeating carbs and sugars. The insulin has knocked on the door of our cells for so long that the cells have begun to ignore the knocks. So we have this overload of energy in our blood stream, but we have no way to process it because our cells stopped opening the door. We become fatter because the insulin starts wrapping our body with layers of unused energy (fat), yet we are tired because our cells are not getting the energy they need. **It's like having an overload of fuel for a car, but instead of the fuel going into the gas tank, it becomes layers of petroleum plastic around the car.** We can't imagine someone choosing a car to become like that, yet this is exactly what we can do to our body.

One way to fight insulin resistance is to eat foods that are low on the GI Scale. Let's not forget: It's not about the foods we can't eat; it's about the foods we can eat. There are so many fabulous foods that we can consume as we forge our way to achieving a healthier body and lifestyle. Our body is wonderfully resilient, and it is never too late to change the path of destruction that we are on. We can start making small changes every day—not just to lose weight, but to transform our life. We can do this for us and for our family. Our children are watching our every move, and they are learning behaviors that will hurt or help them when they are grown. We don't want them to struggle with Type II Diabetes, so let us lead the way to a healthier and fuller life.

GI Scale Chart

More than 70	High
Between 56-69	Moderate
Under 55	Low

Low GI Foods

Food	GI
Peanuts	14
Plain yogurt	14
Soy beans	18
Peas	22
Cherries	22
Grapefruit	25
Black beans	30
Skim milk	32
Whole wheat pasta	37
Apple	38
Pinto beans	39

Moderate GI Foods

Food	GI
Apple Juice	40
Snickers	41
Peach	42
Brown rice	50
Fruit Jam	51
Orange Juice	53
Honey	55
Oatmeal	58
Pineapple	59
Sweet Potato	61
Raisins	64
Whole Wheat Bread	67

High GI Foods

Food	GI
White bread	70
Bagel	72
Watermelon	72
Popcorn	72
French Fries	75
Shredded Wheat	75
Gatorade	78
Corn Flakes	81
Rice Cakes	82
Pretzels	83
Baked Potato	85
Dates	103

Faith
The Power of a Curriculum

Unlike any time in history, our culture has a deluge of information, resources and research at our fingertips. Furthermore, we are more mobile than ever, and we can come face-to-face with experts in any field of study. We have no reason not to better ourselves every day. God wants to provide us with a tailored-made curriculum to help us grow into the fullness of our potential, but we have to give God our attention, energy and time. If our busyness prevents us from learning and growing, we can either limit the time we spend in passive entertainment or we can cut stuff out of our pressing schedule. Yes, it will be a sacrifice, but the sacrifice will be worth it to receive instruction from the Lord.

"Instruct the wise, and they will be even wiser. Teach the righteous, and they will learn even more" (Proverbs 9:9 NLT).

The difficulty about completely adopting someone else's curriculum—whether it be for body, mind our soul—is that it may be hard to integrate into our lifestyle; therefore, it will be impossible to keep for long. We are all designed differently, we live in different environments and we are in different seasons of life. We can use a good curriculum as a springboard, but we will eventually have to cut and add things in order to fit our needs. There are basic rules to staying fit and healthy, but there are many ways to live it out. If we are willing, the Holy Spirit will lead us into a healthy lifestyle that best suits us.

God will use the people, resources and moments in our life to shape us into the masterpiece that He has envisioned for us (Ephesians 2.10). We don't have to worry about trying to pick out our own curriculum–God will bring us into contact with everything we need to succeed for His glory. The Holy Spirit is our Counselor, our Guide, our Teacher and our Coach. He will "guide us into all truth" (John 16.13). We can freely submit to the instruction of the Holy Spirit, knowing that He will equip us to do everything He has planned for our life. He is the Coach of all coaches, and His authority and knowledge have been established before time began. The most wonderful truth is that we have complete and total access to Him at any time–we need only to submit ourselves to His leadership.

*"Now may the God of peace, who through the blood of the eternal covenant brought back from the dead our Lord Jesus, that great Shepherd of the sheep, **equip you with everything good for doing his will**, and may he work in us what is pleasing to him, through Jesus Christ, to whom be glory for ever and ever. Amen" (Hebrews 13.20-21 NIV).*

Chapter 14

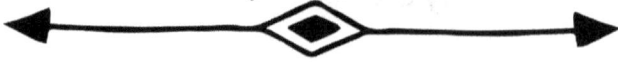

"Then Jesus declared, 'I am the bread of life. Whoever comes to me will never go hungry, and whoever believes in me will never be thirsty'" (John 6.35 NIV).

Fitness
Relaxation

"But whose delight is in the law of the Lord, and who meditates on his law day and night. That person is like a tree planted by streams of water, which yields its fruit in season and whose leaf does not wither—whatever they do prospers" (Psalm 1.2-3 NIV).

Prayer and meditation have little value in a culture that never slows down and is always on the go. Even though watching television, catching a movie and/or reading a good book seems to rest of us physically, we are still filling our minds with the complexities of this world found in the lives of the characters on the show, movie and book. This mental and emotional stimulus is actually affecting our body, and we are not in the total resting state that we imagine. Although there is definitely nothing wrong with enjoying a good show, movie and book, we leave little room in our minds to reflect on our own life and how we are doing. It's hard to take a good look in the mirror when we are so preoccupied with the lives of everyone else—including fictional characters. Most of all, it's hard to consider God's thoughts towards us when our minds are distracted.

"How precious to me are your thoughts, God. How vast is the sum of them." (Psalm 139.17 NIV).

If God's thoughts are precious towards us, shouldn't we take time to receive them? The most relaxing thing we can do for ourselves is to take time to pray to God and to meditate on His Word, the Bible, every day. God is the Source of all that is beautiful, good and perfect, and we can receive from that Source anytime we wish because we have the indwelling of the Holy Spirit through Jesus Christ. Contrary to popular belief, meditation is not the absence of thought; it is the **centering of thoughts on God**—the Source of Life. Prayer and meditation are the single most relaxing, calming and peaceful things we can do for ourselves, yet it is usually the last thing on our list of to-dos.

It's no good sacrificing time staying physically fit if we are spiritually bankrupt. We can have an awesome body and stellar health but still live a defeated, worry-filled life. God wants to talk with us. He wants to fill us with the supernatural gifts of His love, peace and joy. Sometimes we don't even have to say anything. We only need to sit at His feet and find comfort in His presence. God loves us so much that He died for us. He paid a high price to have a relationship with us, and that relationship is too precious to ignore. Not only that, we miss out on the most beautiful love story of all time. The Kingdom of Heaven is literally in our midst, and we can tap into its glory and power whenever we want.

"Nor will people say, 'Here it is,' or 'There it is,' because the kingdom of God is in your midst" (Luke 17.21 NIV).

So let us take special moments every day to spend time with God, praying to Him and meditating on His Word. Let us make a standing appointment daily with Him—not when we rush, reading out the checklist of our needs, but when we can wrap ourselves in the gentle blanket of His love, peace and joy. We can fill our heart, mind and soul with His infinitely wonderful words for us, so we will be empowered to claim victory over the struggles that face us each day. We can read the promises that He has given us in His Word and claim each one of them. And we can remember that we are indeed "wonderfully complex" because His "workmanship is marvelous."

"Thank you for making me so wonderfully complex. Your workmanship is marvelous—how well I know it" (Psalm 139.14 NLT).

Food
Good and Bad Macros

If we eat good foods most of the time, we can splurge on the bad foods once and a while without the sting of guilt. There is nothing wrong with having a dessert or eating a donut with the kids. The problem occurs when we do it so much that it devastates our body and health. Like it has been stated, **we need to enjoy all the foods that we can eat and not focus on the foods we can't eat.** God has given us an amazing array of foods that are tasty and nutritious. We just have to give them a chance. Not only do these foods keep us healthy, they keep us feeling great, as well. When we eat good, healthy foods, our body responds differently than when we eat foods filled with processed carbs and sugars.

The best thing we can do for ourselves when we are doing a food overhaul in our diets is to avoid going out to eat for a while. We can do an "out-to-eat fast" for several weeks or months. Then, when we go to the grocery store, we can creatively fill our carts with healthy and delicious foods. We can see it as a new, fun adventure. Once our palate and body finally detox from the overload of sugars in our diet, we can make healthier choices when we are away from home. It's very easy to fall back into old patterns, and new habits are hard to make. But if we keep at it every day, we will eventually wake up to a healthier lifestyle.

Macros	Good			Bad
	Starchy	**Fibrous**	**Simple**	Fries
Carbs	Potato	Broccoli	Apples	Doughnuts
	Sweet	Spinach	Blueberries	Sodas
	potato	Asparagus	Bananas	Candy
	Yams	Cucumber	Raspberries	White bread
	Squash	Tomatoes	Blackberries	Chips
	Pumpkin	Cauliflower	Nectarines	Pizza
	Brown rice	Brussels	Plums	Sugary
	Lentils	sprouts	Peaches	breakfast
	Couscous	Celery	Pears	cereals
	Quinoa	Onions	Grapefruit	Corn syrup
	Whole	Bell pepper	Pears	Pies
	wheat	Cabbage	Oranges	Cakes
	Whole grain	Kale	Watermelon	Pasta
	Oatmeal	Mushrooms	Cherries	
	Barley	Eggplant	Pineapple	
	Beans	Zucchini	Mango	
	Corn	Carrots	Melon	
	Millet	Green beans		
	Peas	Lettuce		
	Chickpeas			
Proteins	Chicken breast			Pork bacon
	Turkey breast			Deep-fried
	Lean ground turkey			meat
	Swordfish			Chicken
	Salmon			fingers
	Tuna			Fish sticks,
	Crab			Buffalo
	Lobster			wings
	Shrimp			Hamburgers
	Top round steak			Hot dogs
	Top sirloin steak			
	Lean ground beef			
	Buffalo			
	Lean ham			
	Egg whites or substitutes			
	Trout			
	Low-fat cottage cheese			
	Wild-game meat			
	Turkey Bacon			
	Greek Yogurt			
	Cottage Cheese			
	Protein Powders			
Fats	Avocado			Butter
	Sunflower seeds			Lard
	Pumpkin seeds			Mayo
	Cold-water fish			Creamy

	Natural peanut butter Low-fat cheese Low-sodium nuts Olives and olive oil Safflower oil Sunflower oil Flax seed oil Coconut Oil Walnut Oil	sauces Ice cream Shakes

Faith
The Power of Intimacy

"Jesus said to them, 'My food is to do the will of him who sent me and to accomplish his work'" (John 4.34 ESV).

When we accept Jesus to be our Lord and Savior, we begin a new relationship with God. On our own, we are imperfect and unable to connect with a Holy God, but because Jesus died for our sins, giving us His righteousness, the Holy Spirit (God's Spirit) can now enter our lives. This relationship is like a supernatural covenant of marriage—signed with the blood of Jesus Christ. It cannot be broken. However, just like any marriage, we can neglect our relationship with God. Like two ships passing in the night, we can be married and have no interaction. But God wants to have an intimate, personal relationship with us. He wants to interact with us every day and moment-to-moment.

"I love those who love me, and those who seek me find me" (Proverbs 8.17 NIV).

The amazing truth that we can have an intimate relationship with God should fill us with joy. When we are intimate with God, He can give us the power, strength and will to make the changes He wants us to make. We will face difficulty when we begin our journey to achieving a healthier lifestyle, but we can rely on the strength of the Lord. He will fill us with the desire to do His will, and that will become our "food" and our satisfaction. We must have a greater objective than merely looking good and feeling great. We need a higher purpose to our efforts and sacrifices than simply enjoying a better quality of life. God has great plans for us. He created us for a special reason. There is a victory that He wants us to claim and a need He wants us to fill.

When we take time to cultivate our relationship with God, we will discover who we are in Him. If we don't know who we are in God, we won't be able to fulfill our destiny. We can have all the goals in the world, but if they are not rooted in the Vine of Christ, they are done in vain. If our actions are not eternally-minded, they will have no value when we get to heaven. We waste our life when we ignore God. God is our purpose. He is our meaning. He wants to give us power, strength and victory. But most importantly, He wants an intimate relationship with us because He loves us and He enjoys our company. Once we wrap our arms around the Father, we will soon discover that we have found our home.

"I am the vine; you are the branches. If you remain in me and I in you, you will bear much fruit; apart from me you can do nothing" (John 15.5 NIV).

Chapter 15

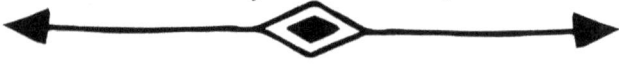

"And the God of all grace, who called you to his eternal glory in Christ, after you have suffered a little while, will himself restore you and make you strong, firm and steadfast" (1 Peter 5.10 NIV).

Fitness
Setting and Achieving Goals

Setting goals is a great way to begin our health and fitness journey. As we continue making healthy lifestyle choices every day, it will take several weeks and/or months to finally see some results. Therefore, we need to set tangible goals that will help motivate us when we are struggling. The **first** thing we can do is jot down our weight and measurements (waist, hips, thighs, etc.) and take before pictures. When we do this, we should instantly put the measurements and pictures away and out of sight. We can get dismayed by what we see and read, and those negative thoughts can fill us with doubt, fear and guilt. But once we lose the weight, those same measurements and pictures will fill us with positive feelings of accomplishment.

The **second** thing we can do is set realistic goals with amazing rewards. For example, if we lose 20 pounds, we can take a trip. Or if we eat healthy for a month, we can splurge on a banana split. Or if we drop a dress size, we can buy two new dresses. Or if we lift 10 more pounds on our bench press, we can go out to eat. Or if we continue our aerobic exercise for 40 minutes, we can take a dip in the gym's Jacuzzi. We can even buy a pair of designer jeans that are one size too small and hang them in our closet to motivate us. Life can be as fun and exciting as we make it, and we can make our fitness and health experience as interesting as we are willing. We can scatter little rewards along the way, giving us the motivation we need to push toward our goal.

The **third** thing we can do is aim towards a future event or occasion. For example, if our class reunion is coming up, we can set that as our goal to get into better shape. Or we can enter and train for a bodybuilding competition. Or we can plan a cruise down the road and aim towards looking great in a swimsuit. Or we can train and race for a marathon. Or we can join a city basketball league and try to win the championship. The possibilities are endless; we just have to get creative, take a risk and give it our all. And once we've accomplished what we set out to achieve, we will be filled with an indescribable sense of satisfaction and triumph.

Food
Cheat Meals

Let's face it: we can't be expected to be perfect all of the time. There are so many delicious "bad" foods out there, and even though we've come to love our healthy foods, we want to be able to splurge sometimes. And so we should be able to have a dessert every now and again. **It's all about self-control, not abstinence**. Remember, we control food; it doesn't control us. Yes, we will have to **get extreme** for a while to reach our goal weight, but once we are maintaining the weight that puts us into our "sweet spot" (with a buffer of 5 pounds), we can start enjoying our cheat meals.

A good standard to keep for food is the **85% and 15% Rule.**

If we eat balanced meals 85% of the week, we can allow for cheat meals 15% of the week.

3 meals x 7 days = 21
21 x .15 (15%) = 3 Cheat Meals a Week

This means we can have 3 cheat meals a week or one cheat day a week. This is exciting news. We can enjoy our favorite "comfort foods," and still embrace a healthy lifestyle. We can look forward to our one full day to enjoy the foods (in moderation) that we've been missing or we can separate our cheat meals and enjoy a cheat meal on special occasions, like a birthday party, or for a date night with someone special. We can thoughtfully plan our cheat meals, so we don't become social stick-in-the-muds, saying no to every cookie offered to us.

We can suck the joy out of life if we are always so strict on ourselves. If we have created a lifestyle of healthy choices, it is okay to stray off the path once in a while. One donut, one scoop of ice cream, one slice of pizza and one serving of pasta won't kill us. In fact, we are not fully living unless we are indulging a little. Remember, **it's about self-control, not abstinence. And we control food; it doesn't control us.**

Faith
The Power of Extreme

"We are hard pressed on every side, but not crushed; perplexed, but not in despair; persecuted, but not abandoned; struck down, but not destroyed" (2 Corinthians 4.8-9 NIV).

Sometimes we need to get physically extreme. We have to say enough is enough, and go all-in to creating a positive difference in our health and fitness. If we don't like the trend our life has taken, it's time to get in gear and make some changes. Changes are hard and they can create fear, and some people may not like the changes we are making, especially the people closest to us. The differences we are creating in our lifestyle will eventually affect them. We must allow them to have their opinions and give them time to adjust. But once they see the positive results from our actions, they may even join our new lifestyle transformation.

There is another extreme that happens to us internally. It's the spiritual extreme that usually no one sees. It's an internal work and very hard to explain to others. People may look at our life and see all the ways that we are blessed, but they may not understand the breaking and reshaping that's happening inside our spirit. God's work inside of each of us is a lonely process. And the end result is always a furthering submission to the Holy Spirit and a transformation into the image of Christ.

*"So all of us who have had that veil removed can see and reflect the glory of the Lord. And the Lord--who is the Spirit--**makes us more and more like him as we are changed into his glorious image**" (2 Corinthians 3.18 NLT).*

God sees the fullness of our life, and He will allow seasons of extreme when He has a goal in sight for us. Out of all the extremes, the spiritual one may be the most difficult to detect because it takes faith. Many times we can't see the plans that God has for us down the road. We don't realize that He has a special "event" for us that will further His Kingdom on earth. But if we are sensitive to the Holy Spirit, we will feel an urgency in our spirit and a readiness for something yet to come, and we will know that it's time for a season of extreme.

So what does extreme accomplish? It helps us to achieve more and go further in less amount of time. It helps us to accomplish goals that force us to stretch and grow. It is a difficult season where we change rapidly with an end goal in sight. It is a short time when we are working full tilt towards the finish line, giving our all to make it to our victory. But it is not something that can be continued for very long, and most often a rest will follow the final push.

When we feel the Holy Spirit prompting a spiritual extreme in us, we need to trust that there is something He is trying to prepare us for. Many Christians miss so many opportunities in life because they are not ready for them. That is why we must daily consult with the

Holy Spirit, asking Him if there is anything today that He wants us to do. We will find that God is providing us everything we need for future victories in pre-ordained moments along the way. We just need to listen, obey and get extreme.

"My sheep listen to my voice; I know them, and they follow me" (John 10.27 NIV).

Conclusion

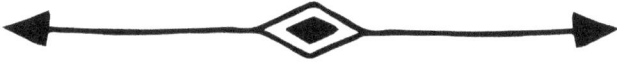

I never set out to write a book like this. Mainly, I didn't think I would ever be *qualified* to relay the information found in these pages. I wanted to write a personal faith-based memoir about competing in a bodybuilding competition. I have always worked out and watched my calories, but I had never set goals higher than simply staying fit and healthy. However, after much confusion and disappointment, I sat down at my desk and stared at the stories, notes and facts I had written and the piles of books I had read. **God wanted more from me, but I didn't know what.** I soon realized that I would have to stretch in order to be obedient to His call on my life for this book. I had to get extreme.

In four months, I trained, competed and placed in a bodybuilding competition. And I studied, tested and became a *Certified Fitness Trainer* and *Specialist in Fitness Nutrition*. Now God called me to write something new with the information that I gained, and He helped motivate me with a dream. A woman came up to me in my dream, and she glowed with peace and joy. She thanked me for the fitness book that I had written. God showed me in this dream that the book was already written; I just needed to type out the pages. Yet I still didn't feel *qualified*, so the next morning God sat me down and had me open my Bible, and I read God's words found in Ezekiel 3.17 (NLT):

*"Son of man, I have appointed you as a **watchman** for Israel. Whenever you receive a message from me, warn people **immediately**."*

I read those words from God and knew that I had just been *made qualified*. There is no greater qualification than when God tells us to do it. I learned after years of obediently communicating God's heart, that no message should be rejected, especially the message of impending destruction. The message that God is giving me is simple: **We are sabotaging the life and purpose that God has given us by the foods we eat and the sedentary activities we do**. The scariest part is that our children are headed down the same path of devastation. We have to put on the brakes now and look at what's happening to God's precious people.

Satan has cunningly created an atmosphere in our culture that is robbing us of our quality of life. And we must speak out and stop the spiral of destruction. We are eating foods that starve us of nutrition, yet encumber us with weight. We are doing activities that sedate our body, diminishing our physical, mental, emotional and spiritual strength. We are anxious, depressed, joyless and fearful all because of our lack of self-control and lack of motivation. Something has to change. Our Kingdom Purpose is buried in the sand, and we are too tired and frustrated to dig it up.

I pray that God uses this book to make that change. I want to see many people like the woman from my dream, filled with peace and joy because they created those small lifestyle changes, saving themselves and their families from destruction. This book has stretched me beyond what I thought was capable, and I have stayed obedient to His call. Now it is your turn. Pray and ask the Holy Spirit to help you. He wants you to live a victorious life for Him. He wants you to have the energy and stamina to dig up your Kingdom Purpose and fulfill it. Don't count the number of times you fall during your health and fitness transformation; count the number of times you take that next step, then the next, then the next.

"Father, Lord, I pray for the people holding this book. I pray that they find the courage and power to change their lives. I pray that they can lean on You for courage and strength when times get tough and they want to give up. Stretch them as You have stretched me. Help them to stay obedient to Your call—not just in health and fitness, but in all areas of life. Show them the abundance of resources available to them that will teach and guide them on their journey to a healthier life. I pray this in the Name Above All Names, Jesus Christ of Nazareth, our Savior and Lord, amen."

6-Week Bible Study
Outline

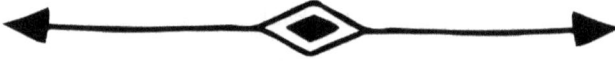

This book can be divided into a 6-week Bible study that meets once a week for an hour and a half. The first week will be an introduction, and the following five weeks will center on the book. The only homework assigned will be to read three chapters and answer the chapter questions for each week.

Assigned Reading and Coursework

Week 1: Read chapters 1-3 and answer chapter questions.

Week 2: Read chapters 4-6 and answer chapter questions.

Week 3: Read chapters 7-9 and answer chapter questions.

Week 4: Read chapters 10-12 and answer chapter questions.

Week 5: Read chapters 13-15 and answer chapter questions.

Week 6: Finish class and continue to be Fearlessly Fit.

Choose Group Discussion Leader

Group discussion is very important to this study. If the Bible study class is large, the Bible study facilitator may not be able to meet with everyone individually. A large class can be divided into smaller groups. The Bible study facilitator will ensure that all the groups are divided equally. Groups are encouraged to meet at the same table with the same individuals each week and assign a group discussion leader. If the Bible study is small, the facilitator can be the group discussion leader.

The first 30 minutes of class will be dedicated to the chapter discussion questions. The group discussion leader can facilitate these questions, allowing each member time to answer if he or she chooses. The members can discuss the assigned chapters and help each other with the material.

The next 30 minutes of class will be dedicated to the Bible lesson for that week. The facilitator can read the Bible lesson for each week and add personal comments and life stories related to the topic. She or he can also engage the group in discussions about the lesson if the group is small. A Bible verse and prayer have been made available and can be read over the group after each lesson.

The final 30 minutes of the class will be dedicated to the Bible lesson discussion questions, which will also be led by the group discussion leader. During this time, people can seek out advice and encouragement from any health professionals or spiritual mentors available in the group.

Introduce Health Professionals

If there are any health and fitness professionals and/or spiritual mentors attending the Bible study, they can volunteer to make themselves available for one-on-one questions during the last 30 minutes of the Bible study each week. These individuals and their professional expertise can be introduced the first day of class. Because time is limited, the volunteer health professionals and spiritual mentors may only be able to give brief advice and encouragement, but their valuable insight is nonetheless appreciated.

Weekly Lifestyle Changes

We will also be making small changes to our lifestyle slowly over the next six weeks. These changes will help us maintain our health and fitness goals for a lifetime. Sudden and drastic changes are very difficult to maintain over the long haul. Instead of changing everything we consider unhealthy all at once, it is better to change one habit a week, which will be #5 of the lesson discussion questions.

Extreme actions tend not stick. Many people will lose a bunch of weight quickly, only to gain it all back. This happens because we are altering our lifestyle to an extreme that we are unable to maintain. Or we cut our food intake so drastically that our body slows down its metabolism because it thinks we are starving. Either way it is better to slowly make changes over a process of time. Even God does not expect us to change everything all at once. Instead, He brings us through a process of going from glory to glory into the image of Christ in degrees, not in an instant.

"And we all, with unveiled face, beholding the glory of the Lord, are being transformed into the same image from **one degree of glory to another.** For this comes from the Lord who is the Spirit" (2 Corinthians 3.18 ESV).

Week 1
Group Ice Breaker Games

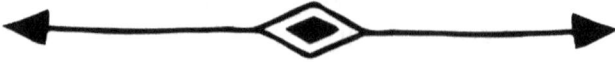

Place your Bible study participants in smaller groups that will be the support system for each member. Make sure these groups are in equal proportions to each other. Assign a discussion leader who is willing to facilitate the chapter and discussion questions for the group. It is good to have ice breaker games the first day of class, so that each group member can get to know the rest of the group and feel comfortable. A list of icebreaker games has been made available, but any fun activity that gets people talking can be implemented.

1. **Commonality:** All the members of the group must find something in common. This commonality can't be something that everyone has (e.g. a mother, a nose, a name). It must be something that is uniquely shared (e.g. all their names have one syllable, they are all born in the same city, they all have two siblings, etc.).

2. **Finding Order:** Each group member must quickly stand and get into alphabetical order by first name without talking to each other. Next get into order by birthday months from January to December. Finally, get into order by height— shortest to tallest.

3. **Fact or Fiction:** Each person of the group will say three things about themselves that the group wouldn't know. Two of those things should be fiction (not true) and one should be fact. The group then needs to guess which thing was fact.

4. **Sentence Maker:** Pick one person to start the sentence by saying a single word. The next person will say the word and add a new word. Then the person after that will repeat both words and add a new word. Go around to each person in the group adding a word until a complete sentence has been made.

5. **Asking Questions:** Each person in the group gets a chance to ask the entire group one question. After one person asks a question, each person takes a turn answering. Then the next person asks a question, and each person in the group answers it until everyone has asked a question. For example, what is your favorite restaurant? Where did you go on your last vacation? What was the last movie or show you watched?

Before starting this week's Bible study, read the introduction out loud to the group on pages 13-16. Discuss how the statistics influence each person's perspective on food and fitness.

Bible Study: Week 1
Imperishable Seed

"For you have been born again, not of perishable seed, but of imperishable, through the living and enduring word of God" (1 Peter 1.23 NIV).

It's important to recognize that gaining a healthy lifestyle means nothing if we are not saved by grace through the blood Jesus shed for us on the cross. What's the point of living in victory for 70 plus years on earth if we are to be separated from God for eternity?

Our relationship or lack of relationship with God will continue beyond our death in this life. Heaven is the presence of God and hell is the absence of God, and the only way we can be in God's presence is through His Son, Jesus. Since God is holy, we cannot have a relationship with Him in our imperfect state. Let's face it: No matter how hard we try, we will never, ever be perfect. The only way we can have a relationship with God is through the grace we receive from the cross.

Jesus came into this earth, exchanged His holiness for our sin and died on the cross, burying our sin in the tomb. The Bible says that Jesus gave His life willingly, but He also had the authority to take His life back up again.

"No one takes it from me, but I lay it down of my own accord. I have authority to lay it down and authority to take it up again. This command I received from my Father" (John 10.18 NIV).

Jesus rose from the grave on the third day, taking back His life. And guess what He left behind? He left behind our sin. Our sin debt has been paid for in full. By faith we stand as righteous people before a Holy God, and we can come before His throne because of the Pierced Lamb of God—the Holy Sacrifice Who has made everything right in the eyes of God.

Once we profess that Jesus is God's Son sent to forgive us our sins and accept Him as our Lord and Savior, an "imperishable seed" is planted in us. This seed represents our eternal life with God in Heaven, and unlike our body, it will never die. Before we delve into the subject of living a healthy lifestyle for God, we must have a relationship with Him. Once we have a relationship with God through Jesus Christ, our future is secure with Him in heaven.

Our relationship with God through Jesus Christ not only secures our souls forever, it also becomes a wellspring of God's strength and power in our lives. If we are unable to tap into God's strength and power on a daily basis, we will struggle with achieving the great things that He has planned for us. God wants us to live in victory, and He will give us everything we need to walk in His power and strength.

"He gives strength to the weary and increases the power of the weak" (Isaiah 40.29 NIV).

If you don't remember a time when you have accepted Jesus as your Lord and Savior, the imperishable seed of God is not within you. But don't fear. God wants you to have a relationship with Him today. That is why He sent His Son, Jesus, to die for you. All you have to do is pray a simple prayer and believe that God sent Jesus to forgive you of all sin and to make you righteous in His eyes.

Please pray the following prayer as a group.

"Dear Jesus, thank You for dying for my sins on the cross. I believe that You shed Your blood to forgive my mistakes and to give me Your righteousness. I want to have a relationship with God today, and I know I can't do it alone. Please come into my life and be my Lord and Savior. I trust that I have been made holy through Your sacrifice and that an imperishable seed has been planted in me. Thank You, Jesus, for dying for me. I pray this in Your name, amen."

If you have prayed this prayer for the first time, you are now a child of God. God's Spirit, the Holy Spirit, now dwells inside of the imperishable seed that has been planted in you. The Holy Spirit will help guide you on your walk of faith as you learn to listen to His voice. Also, God has given you His Word, the Bible, to be a light, guiding your steps every day. God wants to deepen His relationship with you, so pray to Him everyday, so you can get to know Him even more.

Verse and prayer for breaking strongholds:

"The weapons we fight with are not the weapons of the world. On the contrary, they have divine power to demolish strongholds" (2 Corinthians 10.4 NIV).

"Father, we bind and break the devil's strongholds on our lives. We pray by the power of the resurrection spirit and Jesus' blood shed on the cross that every tool of the enemy is rendered powerless. We boldly claim by the authority afforded to us as righteous children of God that the devil's footholds are demolished and his evil schemes are exposed and decreed useless. We believe that we have the victory through Jesus Christ to overcome every struggle and temptation that we face. We pray this in Jesus' name, amen."

Discussion Questions:

1. What are some strongholds that you may have in the area of food and fitness? Discuss with the group any area that you may be struggling.

2. Discuss how God has helped you during a time of struggle. Did He send a book, person, sermon, song and/or movie in your path that has encouraged you?

3. Do you have any health related problems that are in your family or in your life personally? How can this 6-week study help you to overcome those difficulties?

4. Discuss the health goals that the Holy Spirit is prompting you to achieve during the next 6 weeks with your group.

5. Discuss one healthy habit that you will be adding to your daily routine this week.

Week 2

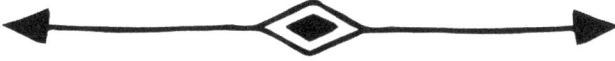

1. Which body type do you think describes you the most? Are you a combination of two body types?

2. How does knowing your body type help you to understand your body more and better achieve your health goals?

3. According to your body type, what would be your macronutrient breakdown?

4. Which macronutrient do you tend to favor most— proteins, carbohydrates or fats?

5. Between 1-10 (1 being no struggle and 10 being extreme struggle) how much would you say you struggle with self-control? How has this affected your health?

6. How many hours per week do you exercise? Would you like to increase the length or the difficulty level of your work out routine?

7. What is your Body Mass Index (BMI)? Do you want to decrease, increase or maintain your BMI?

8. How can you incorporate more strength training exercises into your schedule?

9. Was there a description of the macronutrients (protein, carbohydrates and fats) that surprised you?

10. What can you do today to begin making changes to your lifestyle to promote healthier results?

Before we continue the Bible study, make sure that all the Bible study members download a calorie counter app to their smart phones. If they do not have an app on their phone, they can do it online or keep a food journal.

Bible Study: Week 2
Sling or Sword

"As the Philistine moved closer to attack him, David ran quickly toward the battle line to meet him. Reaching into his bag and taking out a stone, he slung it and struck the Philistine on the forehead. The stone sank into his forehead, and he fell facedown on the ground. So David triumphed over the Philistine with a sling and a stone; without a sword in his hand, he struck down the Philistine and killed him. David ran and stood over him. He took hold of the Philistine's sword and drew it from the sheath. After he killed him, he cut off his head with the sword" (1 Samuel 17.48-51 NIV).

Many people believe that the sling killed Goliath, but another interpretation suggests that the sling only knocked him out. It is Goliath's own sword that David used to kill him and to chop off his head. However, when Goliath became unconscious from the stone that David slung into his skull, his fate was sealed. In probably less than 30 seconds, David had the sword unsheathed and was holding Goliath's head.

The truth is that David could not have killed Goliath without the sling taking the enemy down first. David needed both the sling and the sword to conquer Goliath, and he needed to use them in a specific order: first the sling and then the sword. In this same way, we will also fight enemies that are stronger, mightier and bigger than us. And God will equip us with two weapons to claim victory: the sling and the sword.

"Take the helmet of salvation and the sword of the Spirit, which is the word of God" (Ephesians 6.17 NIV).

The sword can be compared to the Word of God, the Holy Bible of Truth. When we battle the "Goliaths" in our lives, including our weight and health, we must read our Bibles and apply the promises found in the verses to claim our triumph. God's Word will always lead to our greater victory in His Kingdom. However, we may come across enemies in our lives that are rooted so deep and their influence is so strong that we must get additional support to defeat them. These additional resources of support can be compared to slings. For example, this health book we are reading is a sling in our lives, helping us to claim victory in our health.

Many well meaning Christians will say that all we need is the Sword of the Spirit (God's Word) to overcome strongholds in our lives. Of course, we cannot defeat anything without the Bible, but many times we need supplemental Christian resources to help "knock out" our foes first. Christian books, movies, music, counselors, sermons, classes, groups, etc. are all excellent "slings" that we can use along side our Bibles to defeat the strong enemies in our lives. The bigger the problem, the more slings we need to get.

"Then Saul dressed David in his own tunic. He put a coat of armor on him and a bronze helmet on his head. David fastened on his sword over the tunic and tried walking around, because he was not used to them. 'I cannot go in these,' he said to Saul, 'because I am not used to them.' So he took them off" (1 Samuel 17.38-39 NIV).

King Saul tried to give David his armor and sword to beat Goliath, but David said, "I cannot go in these because I am not used to them." The truth is that we all have our own battles to fight, and many times we are not yet able to kill Goliath using someone else's interpretation of what we should do. We first have to claim God's power in our lives and knock the giant out with a sling. It may take many slings and many shots to bring Goliath down, but with God's help we will eventually get him to the ground. And once Goliath's stronghold in our lives has been knocked out, we can finally wield God's Holy Word and cut him off for good.

To beat the giants in our lives, there is a process that we must walk through first, and our health is no different. We can surround ourselves for a time with resources that will help us claim victory in our health and fitness, and we can rely on the eternal Truth found in the Bible to bring the deadly blow. As we weaken the strongholds in our lives by using the slings that God has given, we grow stronger in our hope and confidence in the Lord and His Word. God's Word is alive and active, and God's Spirit will pour from the pages and into our situations. But we need to do our part and be prepared with our slings for battle.

"For the word of God is alive and active. Sharper than any double-edged sword, it penetrates even to dividing soul and spirit, joints and marrow; it judges the thoughts and attitudes of the heart" (Hebrews 4.12 NIV).

Verse and prayer for claiming victory:

"All Scripture is God-breathed and is useful for teaching, rebuking, correcting and training in righteousness, so that the servant of God may be thoroughly equipped for every good work" (2 Timothy 3.16-17 NIV).

"Father, we want to finally beat the Goliath of unhealthiness in our lives. Help us to come to battle prepared with our sling of resources. We know that Your Word will have the final blow, so we want to read as much of the Bible as we can, filling our heart, soul and mind with the truth and promises found in its pages. Today, we claim the victory over our giants. We know that God is fighting for us, and Jesus has already overcome the world. We pray this in Jesus' name, amen."

Discussion Questions:

1. Discuss any "Goliaths" in your lives that you have been battling without a "sling."

2. Discuss what "sling" or resources you can add to your life to weaken your enemies?

3. Discuss a time in the past where you used a "sling" to help you accomplish your goal and overcome difficulty. How was it helpful in aiding your success?

4. Make a list of any resources that you can add to your health journey during the next 6 weeks.

5. Discuss one healthy habit that you will be adding to your daily routine this week?

Week 3

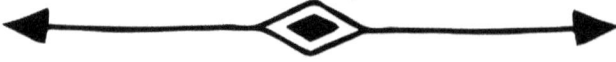

1. What is your resting heart rate? What implications does it have on your health?

2. What is your Basal Metabolic Rate (BMR)? How will knowing your BMR help you to adjust how you eat in order to improve your body mass index?

3. How many pounds would you like to lose or gain within a year?

4. If a pound is 3,500 calories, how many calories will you have to drop from your BMR each day to reach your goal weight?

5. Why is it better to lose weight over the long run, instead of losing all of it too quickly?

6. Have you ever found yourself speaking negative words over your life? What can you do to start speaking positive words of truth into your struggle and situation?

7. According to your age and gender, what is your target heart rate and what is your max heart rate? Have you ever experience a time when you believe that you may have hit your max heart rate during strenuous activity?

8. Do you prefer anaerobic or aerobic exercise more? How can you integrate both types of exercise into your daily schedule?

9. According to your body type, how many calories will you dedicate your diet to each macronutrient—protein, carbohydrates and fats?

10. Nutrition labels on foods are broken down in grams, so it is good to convert our calories from each macronutrient into grams. What is the breakdown of grams for each macronutrient in your diet?

Bible Study: Week 3
Painful Labor, Painful Toil

To the woman: "I will greatly multiply your sorrow and your conception; **In pain you shall bring forth children**; Your desire *shall be* for your husband, And he shall rule over you" (Genesis 3.16 NKJV).

To the man: "Cursed *is* the ground for *your sake*; **In toil you shall eat *of* it** All the days of your life" (Genesis 3.17 NKJV).

Adam and Eve sinned and could not be in God's presence in the Garden of Eden anymore because they were no longer His perfect creation. God is holy, and He can only dwell with that which is holy. Adam and Eve represent all of humanity and our choice to walk away from the holiness and perfection of God. We separated ourselves from God because of our free will choice to sin, so God allowed the earth (also His perfect creation) to be cursed for our own sake, enabling us to see our need for Redemption and a Savior by faith.

God told Eve that she would have painful labor, and He told Adam that he would have painful toil. Both of these "pains" symbolize that men and women will have sorrows, pain and work in this life. But God allowed these things for our own good. Our sorrows, pain and work cause us to reach out for Jesus and long for a relationship with God even though we can't see Him.

The pains and sorrows of this earth force us to understand our lack and realize that we need a savior and our fallen world needs redemption. If this life was easy, we may be tempted to think we don't need a relationship with God, and we would continue in our separation for eternity. Jesus died for our sins, though, and now we can be reconciled back to God even in our sinful state, but we must see our need for Him.

Once we die on this earth, the relationship we have with God through Jesus Christ continues, and we will stand in God's presence in heaven once more--a perfect creation because of Jesus' sacrifice. If we don't have a relationship with God through Jesus Christ, that lack of relationship will continue after we die, and we will be in the absence of God's presence, which is what we call hell. Praise God for the sorrows of this earth or none of us would call out the name of Jesus and claim His salvation.

Everything in this life takes work. The expression "no pain, no gain," rings true not only in the gym, but in every aspect of existence on earth. God's promises, the goals that we set and the dreams that we have will all take work. God does give us seasons of rest, but most of the time staying obedient to God will hurt a little bit, and sometimes it will even hurt a lot. Managing our health is no different. If we are not working at staying healthy, our health is probably on the decline.

The word, *Eden*, actually means "pleasure." In heaven, we will be surrounded by the pleasure of the

Lord, and it will be the most amazing experience ever. However, on earth to be surrounded by too much pleasure can leave devastating results. When the pleasure of our lives outweighs the work of our lives, we will experience many problems. For example, the pleasure of overeating and the pleasure of eating too many rich foods can cause us to gain excess weight. The pleasure of passive entertainment and the pleasure of physical inactivity can cause our muscles to atrophy. These pleasures that should give us small, refreshing rests from our work have become large portions of our day.

The scary part is that people have become so distracted by these fleeting pleasures that they no longer see their need for Jesus. It's like we are trying to create our own "Eden" on this earth—a place of pleasure that does not contain the presence of God. But only our relationship with God through the sacrifice of Jesus Christ will provide us with the purest form of pleasure—one that encourages us and builds us up; instead of only masking the pain and sorrows of this life. We can be encouraged, though. Yes, this life has pain and sorrows and it takes work, but Jesus came into this earth to bear those sorrows with us. Jesus says in Matthew 11.28-30 (NIV):

"Come to me, all you who are weary and burdened, and I will give you rest. Take my yoke upon you and learn from me, for I am gentle and humble in heart, and you will find rest for your souls. For my yoke is easy and my burden is light."

A yoke is a symbol of work, so we will have work in this life, but we won't have to do it alone. The yoke was worn by oxen, and the oxen are always counted in pairs in the Bible. When we put on our yoke, we know that Jesus is wearing His right along side of us. In fact, we are yoked together because of His grace for us and our faith in Him. God left His throne to come to this earth in order to wear a yoke with us and experience the sorrow and pain of this life too. We are not alone. Jesus walks down the same dusty roads and toils the same hard ground with us.

In fact, the Book of Isaiah prophesies that the Messiah will take our pain and bear our suffering. Yes, this life is hard and it takes work, but the ultimate suffering and pain was taken by Jesus Christ on the Cross. We all deserve to be separated from God because of our sin, but Jesus took our sin and separation when He died on the cross. He overcame sin and death when He rose from the grave on the third day. Now we can trust that our suffering, pain and sorrow will have an end. We will someday be reconciled to the Garden of Eden, but now sin will no longer hinder us because grace and faith have filled the gap of separation. And we can enjoy the pleasure of the Lord for eternity in His presence.

"Surely he took up our pain and bore our suffering, yet we considered him punished by God, stricken by him, and afflicted" (Isaiah 53.4 NIV).

Verse and prayer while committing to work:

"May the favor of the Lord our God rest on us; establish the work of our hands for us-- yes, establish the work of our hands" (Psalm 90.17 NIV).

"Father God, we claim right now that You bless the works of our hands. Establish all that we do in obedience to Your will for Your glory. We know that our work can be hard, but we are comforted to know that You are walking right beside us. Thank You, God, for sending Jesus to bear the weight of this broken world with us. Thank You for allowing Yourself to be yoked to us. We praise Your name for the sorrows and pain in our lives because they have helped us to see our need for a Savior. We give You the effort of our hands, God. We pray that Jesus redeems our work and multiplies our efforts. We pray this in Jesus' name, amen."

Discussion Questions:

1. Discuss in areas in your life that you may have been indulging in too many pleasures.

2. Discuss any work that you have been avoiding because it sounded too hard or too painful to commit to.

3. Discuss how knowing that we ultimately will have a life in Christ that is free from suffering, pain and sorrow in heaven encourages you in the work of this life.

4. Look back over your Body Mass Index, your resting heart rate and your Basal Metabolic Rate. Discuss with your group any details that you are willing to share about where your health needs improvement.

5. Discuss one healthy habit that you will be adding to your daily routine this week.

Week 4

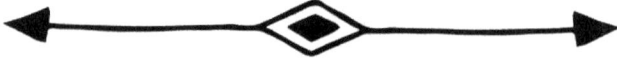

1. If you had to choose an exercise that you enjoy most, which one would it be? How can you fit that exercise into your daily schedule?

2. How do you think having a regular workout routine will benefit your health other than simply losing weight?

3. How would you categorize your energy level at work: Sedentary, lightly active, active or very active? How does this affect your health goals?

4. What is your Total Daily Energy Expenditure (TDDE)?

5. How can obedience help you reach your health and fitness goals?

6. In your own words, describe High Intensity Internal Training (HIIT). How can you integrate more of HIIT into your daily schedule without taking too much time from other responsibilities?

7. What are your feelings about strength training? What are some ways you can start adding strength training into your schedule?

8. Explain the importance of the Glycemic Index. How does the information you gain affect how you eat?

9. Fiber is very important to any healthy diet. What fibrous foods do you enjoy most and how can you integrate more of them into your schedule?

10. Has there been a time in your life when you believed God was putting you through a spiritual contraction? How did you get through the strengthening process? What was the end result?

Bible Study: Week 4
The Useless Loincloth

"So I went to the Euphrates and dug it out of the hole where I had hidden it. But now it was rotting and falling apart. The loincloth was good for nothing" (Jeremiah 13.7 NLT).

God taught Jeremiah a lengthy lesson about taking advantage of God's blessings. Jeremiah lived in a time much like today when the people were so blessed by the hand of God that they forgot the Source of their blessing. God warned the people over and over again to stay obedient to Him, but they didn't listen. Eventually, God's people would become so corrupted that the countries surrounding them would overtake them. God's children became useless to the Kingdom of Heaven, and their nation fell apart. They had forsaken God, and it would take hundreds of years for God's people to reestablish their nation once more.

God told Jeremiah to walk to the Euphrates River to bury a loincloth. This definitely seemed like a strange request, but God needed to give us a visual image of what was happening to His children. Jeremiah must have felt that carrying a loincloth and burying it in the rocks didn't seem like much of a calling from God. But that's the important key to being used by God: We obey even when we don't quite understand. Unlike most of God's children, Jeremiah was willing to be used…even if it meant carrying underwear.

Instead of being worn like it was created to be, the loincloth was carried and buried in a hole. Jeremiah went back home and waited for further instructions from God. After a time, God had Jeremiah walk back to the Euphrates River and dig up the loincloth. However, the loincloth fell apart and became "good for nothing." This is precisely what happens to Christians when they don't allow themselves to be used by God. We hide from God in the shelter of His blessings in our lives, and we fall apart because we are not being used for the purposes that He designed us.

Much like the loincloth, our body was designed to be used. If we allow our body to be carried from one place to the next and then plop it down in front of the TV or computer for hours, it will begin to fall apart. It is interesting that exercise is actually considered the only genuine "fountain of youth" that is available to us. When we use our body in consistent physical activities, we are actually strengthening our bones, muscles, joints, lungs, veins, etc. Yes, we can injure ourselves while doing activity, but the alternative to an active lifestyle can be much worse. Lifestyle related diseases are the main cause of death in our society today. Our body was designed to be used and to stay active.

The difficulty we face when trying to stay active is that our culture has created a lifestyle that keeps us from exercise. Technology has greatly improved our lives, but it has also stolen our ability to move. Cars, phones, Internet, washing machines, refrigerators, etc. are all wonderful blessings, but they have greatly decreased our physical activities. Today, we have to <u>choose</u> to stay active. We have to choose to walk, choose to go to the gym, choose to lift weights, choose to ride our bikes. Staying active is no longer a circumstance that is forced on us. Rather, we have to obediently make a choice to be good stewards of our body and commit to getting the appropriate amount of exercise.

The same goes for every aspect of our lives: our bodies, minds, relationships and faith all must be used and moved by God. Nothing ever stays stagnate. We are either pressing forward or falling back. Yes, rest is involved in moving forward with God because it is a necessary part of our growth. There is nothing wrong with taking shelter in the safety of the Lord after a season of difficulty.

"The Lord is my rock, my fortress and my deliverer; my God is my rock, in whom I take refuge, my shield and the horn of my salvation, my stronghold" (Psalm 18.2 NIV).

However, finding safety in the shelter of the Lord after being used by Him is a lot different than the example of Jeremiah's loincloth. The loincloth was so sheltered in the rock that it began to rot. We want to be used by God. We want to be so worn out by our service for Him at the end of our lives that we can't wait for heaven. The other alternative is that we stay sheltered in His blessings—always hiding from being used for His service—that we literally become "good for nothing" for His Kingdom. But that's not what God wants for our lives. He wants us to be like Paul who at the end of his life knew that he had done everything that the Lord had called him to, and he had a crown of righteousness waiting for him in heaven.

"I have fought the good fight, I have finished the race, I have kept the faith. Now there is in store for me the crown of righteousness, which the Lord, the righteous Judge, will award to me on that day—and not only to me, but also to all who have longed for his appearing" (2 Timothy 4.7-8 NIV).

Verse and Prayer for being used by God:

"For we are God's handiwork, created in Christ Jesus to do good works, which God prepared in advance for us to do" (Ephesians 2.10 NIV).

"Father, help us not to feel condemned. We want to humble ourselves to Your correction and stay obedient to how You are moving in our lives at this moment. We want to be used for Your service. We not only want to keep our bodies active for You, we want to make an effort in all the areas of our lives. God, use us for the special purpose that You have created for us before our birth. We want our lives to impact this generation for Your Kingdom and Your glory. We pray this in Jesus' name, amen."

Discussion Questions:

1. Discuss how technological advances have greatly limited your ability to stay involved in physical activities?

2. Discuss how you can cut some sedentary activities from your schedule, so you may have more time to stay active.

3. Discuss any call of service from God that you may have been avoiding. How can God use you for His service in His Kingdom?

4. Write a work out plan for your week. Discuss with your group the activities you plan on implementing into your schedule.

5. Discuss one healthy habit that you will be adding to your daily routine this week.

Week 5

Chapter Questions 10-12

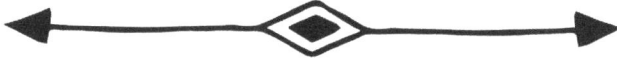

1. What's the difference between slow-twitch and fast-twitch muscle fibers? Which muscle fibers do you use most in your work out routine?

2. Why is it important to tear muscles down in order to build them back up? How is this truth relevant in our spiritual lives?

3. According to your body type, what kind of exercise routine will suit you best? Do you follow this stereotype or work beyond it?

4. Why is it important to reach all your macronutrient goals each day? How can consuming too much of any one macronutrient be a hindrance to your health?

5. What are some of your most favorite "comfort foods"? What are some healthier options that you've learned to love?

6. Many restaurants serve large portions that exceed the recommended portion size. How does this influence how we eat when we are away from home?

7. What are your thoughts about "grazing"? How can you add healthier snacks in between your regular meal times?

8. Are you aware of any muscle imbalance in your body? Are there in previous injuries or current ailments that need to be considered when creating an exercise routine?

9. Stretching is very important for a healthy body. How often do you stretch? Is there a way that you can add stretching to your daily schedule?

10. Water is extremely important to the health of your body. What plan can you create to ensure that you drink the recommended amount of water each day?

Bible Study: Week 5
Bread for Stones

"The tempter came to him and said, 'If you are the Son of God, tell these stones to become bread'" (Matthew 4.3 NIV).

All of God's children are called to the wilderness for various seasons. The wilderness of our lives is what builds our faith and keeps us clinging onto God. Jesus, though He was the perfect Son of God, experienced the wilderness for forty days as an example to us. Since Jesus obediently allowed God to lead Him into the desert, we have no excuse to run away when the Holy Spirit leads us to the desert of difficulty in our own lives.

There are two types of wilderness experiences. The first wilderness experience is brought on by circumstances that are out of our control. Whether they are caused by the repercussions of our own actions or by the actions of others, we have no way of avoiding the desert before us. The second wilderness experience is brought on by circumstances that we obediently walk into. Much like Jesus obediently walked into the desert to be tempted, God will call us into situations that are difficult because they test and refine us.

When Jesus fasted for forty days, He allowed God to test and refine Him. His time in the desert is an example of the second type of wilderness experience because He obediently withheld food from His body, thereby creating a difficult situation in His life through obedience. During this difficulty, Satan tempted Jesus three times. The first temptation that Jesus experienced was to turn stones into bread. This temptation is seemingly harmless. Why wouldn't Jesus want to feed Himself? He was starving. The only problem is that at the moment God was giving Jesus stones, not bread, and to change what God was presenting to Him would be an act of disobedience to the will of God.

These stones represent two things. The first thing they represent is difficulty. It is the difficulties in life that strengthen us, and many times God will lead us into difficult situations to build us up. If Jesus would have turned the stones into bread as Satan tempted Him to do, He would have circumvented what God was trying to accomplish in His life during the wilderness experience.

When we run away from the difficult situations in our own lives, we too will circumvent what God is trying to accomplish in us. To believe that God always wants our lives to be happy, easy and comfortable is to believe a lie. Indeed, God wants to produce joy and hope in us, but He wants them to be rooted in His Spirit in us and not our natural circumstances. God will lead us through difficulty on earth because He is molding us into the amazing design He created us to be.

If all God wanted for us was His salvation, He would take us straight to heaven once we accept Jesus Christ as Lord and Savior. However, God wants more than our salvation, which is why He keeps us on earth until His will in our lives is accomplished. He wants to develop us into the mature Christians that we will be for eternity. This life is much like a womb. We are growing the imperishable seed in us before we die on this earth and are born into the Kingdom of Heaven.

The stones also represent the foundation of Jesus. Jesus is many times compared to a stone in both the Old and New Testaments. This stone signifies that our foundation in God is always Jesus. He must be our rock in every situation and circumstance if we want to live a life pleasing to God.

"So this is what the Sovereign Lord says: 'See, I lay a stone in Zion, a tested stone, a precious cornerstone for a sure foundation; the one who relies on it will never be stricken with panic'" (Isaiah 28.16 NIV).

However, Jesus also calls Himself the "Bread of Life." Bread is our basic staple of nourishment in our lives. "Breaking bread" with others is also symbolic of fellowship and community.

"Then Jesus declared, 'I am the bread of life. Whoever comes to me will never go hungry, and whoever believes in me will never be thirsty'" (John 6.35 NIV).

What we find is that Jesus is both the Stone and the Bread, but there is an order of receiving Him. We must first make Jesus the foundation of our lives through obedience before we can completely taste His goodness. Many people want all the goodness of the Lord, but they don't want to obey Him. They run away from the difficulties of the wilderness and wonder why they are not growing spiritually. But we can't have the Bread unless we first accept the Stone. Jesus must be the foundation of our lives, and that means we obey when He calls us into difficulty. Once we learn obedience, we can taste the goodness of the Lord.

"Taste and see that the LORD is good; blessed is the one who takes refuge in him" (Psalm 34.8 NIV).

Verse and prayer while enduring hardships:

"For our light and momentary troubles are achieving for us an eternal glory that far outweighs them all" (2 Corinthians 4.17 NIV).

"Father, help us to not run away from hardships. Learning to achieve a healthy lifestyle will not be easy at first, but we know You will give us the strength we need to overcome and achieve victory. We want You to be the foundation of our lives, so we will endure the struggle for a time, knowing that we will be rewarded with a higher quality of life in You. Thank You for refining us into the image of Jesus. We know that You have us on earth for a purpose and that none of the difficulties we endure goes in vain. You are using all the circumstances of life to make us into the spiritual powerhouses You created us to be. We want to make

You our foundation, so we can taste Your goodness. We pray this in Jesus' name, amen."

Discussion Questions:

1. Discuss a step of obedience that you have been avoiding.

2. Discuss a struggle that God asked you to walk through in the past and how it strengthened your faith.

3. Discuss any food or fitness related difficulties that you are currently facing.

4. Write down any negative attitudes you may be carrying that prevent you from living a healthy lifestyle. Cross out each negative attitude on your list and replace it with a word of victory.

5. Discuss one healthy habit that you will be adding to your daily routine this week.

Week 6

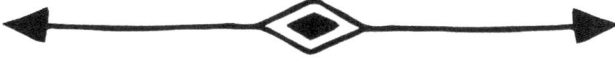

1. Would you ever consider hiring a personal trainer for a season? Why or why not?

2. What is insulin resistance? How can an exercise program prevent insulin resistance, which can lead to diabetes?

3. What are some low glycemic foods that you already enjoy?

4. Today we are blessed to have so many resources at our disposal? Detail some resources that you have chosen to help you on your health journey.

5. What are some ways that you can implement relaxation into your schedule beyond passive entertainment?

6. How can meditating on God and His Word help you to relax?

7. Detail a time when the Holy Spirit gave you peace in the middle of a struggle or sorrow?

8. What are some ways you can spoil yourself when you meet your personal health goals?

9. What are your thoughts on cheat meals? Would you rather have three cheat meals throughout the week or one cheat day?

10. Changing the health of your body may take work but getting "extreme" for a little while can be worth it. What can you do to get extreme, so you can reach your health goals?

Bible Study: Week 6
Abstinence vs. Self-Control

Abstinence is necessary for people who have lost all self-control in certain areas of life. God may place parameters of abstinence around people for a time in order to protect them from temptations that they are unable to withstand. Unlike the Ten Commandments, these specific convictions that the Lord places on people are many times not for everyone. They are for individuals in their unique weaknesses, circumstances and backgrounds.

For example, the Holy Spirit may convict someone to stay away from alcohol if he or she always drinks to drunkenness. Or the Holy Spirit may convict someone to not bring home sweets or snacks if he or she continues to overeat them. These convictions are not for everyone; rather, they are designed specifically for a person who is struggling to resist a certain temptation and lacks self-control.

The goal in our lives, however, is to be like Jesus. He was so in tuned and submitted to the will of God on a second-to-second basis, that he brought His holiness to every situation. He didn't needs rigid parameters because His longing was always to do the will of the Father. He was unaffected by the things of this world, so He had complete freedom from the Father to do as He pleased. Jesus was always about His Father's business—no matter who He was with, what He was doing and where He was going. He influenced the people and circumstances around Him for good, so He could be trusted anywhere, with anything and with everyone.

"For I have come down from heaven not to do my will but to do the will of him who sent me" (John 6.38 NIV).

This freedom seemed to surprise Jesus' disciples and the religious leaders of the time. The disciples found Jesus talking to a Samaritan woman who obviously had a sexual promiscuous past since she had five husbands. For the Son of God to be seen talking by Himself to this woman must have been a real shock to the disciples. But that was the thing about Jesus. He could be trusted, so He didn't need the strict parameters that religious people of the day embraced. He influenced this woman for good, and He remained holy and unaffected by her sins.

"Just then his disciples returned and were surprised to find him talking with a woman. But no one asked, 'What do you want?' or 'Why are you talking with her?'" (John 4.27 NIV).

Today, God has lifted the stringent laws of the holiness that He gave to the Jews because now we have freedom in Christ by grace. This doesn't mean we do whatever we want to please ourselves because of grace. It means that by grace we can do what God desires in order to accomplish His will in our lives.

When we have strict parameters in our lives, we don't have to rely on the Holy Spirit. These strict parameters cause us to rely on rules rather than on God's movements in our lives. We may seem righteous in our own eyes, but our rigidity will cause us to miss out on the great plans God has for us.

For example, if we say we are never going to eat desserts, we may never overeat sweets, but we miss out on cultivating our relationship with the Lord in the area of food. If we give ourselves freedom to enjoy desserts but stay sensitive to the Holy Spirit's leading before eating, we are empowered to stay in contact with Him through every decision in our lives—big or small. The Holy Spirit may say, "Yes, you can have that dessert" or "No, that is not for you today."

Relying on God keeps us in constant communication with Him for every decision in our lives. We never know what God will do through our complete reliance on Him. God may have a great plan for our lives that begins with a shared dessert with a fellow Believer. But we won't discover it if we have forced a strict rule of abstinence in our lives.

The truth of that matter is that it's not about self-control; it's about God-control. We need to be aware of our weakness and allow God to lay out His parameters for areas in which we stumble, but we can boldly walk in freedom in the other areas of life to which God has given us strength. We also need to be very careful not to push our unique convictions on everyone else (this does not include the Ten

Commandments). God may tell one person that he or she should avoid coffee for a season, but that doesn't mean everyone around that person needs to be hammered with the same conviction. It's easy to transfer our personal convictions onto everyone else, but we must realize that God has a specific plan for each one of us that calls for individualized parameters to lead us to where we need to be. The Holy Spirit is doing a personal work in each of us, so comparing ourselves to others will only confuse the situation and put unnecessary rules on people.

In John 21.18-23 after the resurrection, Jesus tells Peter that when Peter becomes old, he will be killed and his death would glorify God. When Peter heard the news about his death, he instantly turned to John and said, "What about him?" Jesus did not indulge Peter in that comparison. He simply said, "If I want him to remain alive until I return, what is that to you? You must follow me." Little did Peter know that John would have to stay alive, so he could write the Book of Revelations—the final book of the Bible.

We learn from this story that is so easy to compare ourselves to others, but what God is doing in another person's life should not affect our submission to what God is doing in our own life. Comparisons will rob us of joy if we let them. God gives freedom to people according to their weaknesses, strengths, designs and callings. Someone may have a freedom that we don't have, but they will also have a parameter that we don't have. We need to be concerned about what God is doing in us and not what God is doing in the lives of others, knowing that when we do our own part, we help all the parts of God's Kingdom. Only then can we be perfectly fit in our own lives and as a whole with other Believers.

"He makes the whole body **fit together perfectly**. As each part does its own special work, it helps the other parts grow, so that the whole body is healthy and growing and full of love" (Ephesians 4.16 NLT).

Verse and prayer for claiming God-control:

"But we are citizens of heaven, where the Lord Jesus Christ lives. And we are eagerly waiting for him to return as our Savior" (Philippians 3.20 NLT).

"Father, we know that we are citizens of heaven who are only on this earth for a short time. Help us to desire Your will above all things. We want to fulfill the great purposes that You have created for us since before time began. We want to lean on You in every area of life, including our fitness and food. Help us to be more reliant on You, so we can learn to walk in the freedom of Your grace. We don't want to be regulated by laws; rather, we want to be moved in the spirit to please God and obey His commands in our lives. We pray this in Jesus' name, amen."

Discussion Questions:

1. What are some strict parameters that God has placed in your life?

2. Have you ever experienced a time in your life where God gave you freedom in an area that you once struggled?

3. Have you ever forced your personal convictions on someone else? Did this cause tension in your relationship?

4. How can relying on God in the area of food and fitness help you to better achieve your goals?

5. Discuss one healthy habit that you will be adding to your daily routine this week.

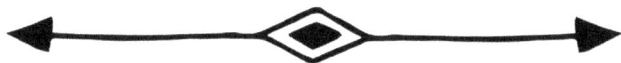

You can also check out Alisa's other health and fitness book, *Fearlessly Fit at Home*, which includes an at home workout program. If you love this book, please write a review. And discover Alisa's many fiction and non-fiction books on Amazon or her blog: www.alisahopewagner.com.

www.ingramcontent.com/pod-product-compliance
Lightning Source LLC
Chambersburg PA
CBHW071119280326
41935CB00010B/1064